FROM DISCOMFORT TO RELIEF

NATURAL REMEDIES AND SELF-CARE PRACTICES FOR PLUGGED DUCTS

Alice Brendan

Introduction 4

Chapter 1: Understanding 6

Plugged Ducts: 6

Chapter 2: Natural Remedies for Plugged Ducts: Healing from Within
.... 19

Chapter3: Breaking the Cycle: Preventing Plugged Ducts Before They
Happen 31

Chapter 4: Healing Hands: Massage Techniques for Plugged Ducts 44

Chapter 5: Cultivating Inner Peace Mindful Practices for Plugged ... 55

Chapter 6: Support Systems: Building a Strong Network for Plugged
Duct Recovery 68

Chapter 7: Overcoming Challenges: Strategies for Dealing with
Stubborn Plugged Ducts 80

Chapter 8: The Healing Power of Nature: Harnessing Earth's
Remedies for Plugged Duct Relief 94

Chapter 9: Beyond the Pain: Rediscovering Comfort and Ease with
Plugged Ducts Beyond the Pain 105

Chapter 10: The Path to Healing: Embracing Natural Remedies for
Plugged Duct Relief 119

Chapter 11: Healing from Within: Natural Remedies and Self-Care
Practices for Plugged Ducts Healing from Within 133

Chapter 12: The Power of Self-Healing: Finding Relief from Plugged
Ducts Naturally 148

Chapter 13: The Road to Recovery: Strategies for Clearing Plugged
Ducts and Finding Relief The Road to Recovery 160

Chapter 14: Empowering Yourself with Knowledge 173

Conclusion 177

Biography 178

Printed in the United States of America.

For more information, or to book an event, contact :
(Email & Website)

Book design by (Alice Brendan)
Cover design by Alice Brendan)

Introduction

Welcome, dear readers, to "From Discomfort to Relief: Natural Remedies and Self-Care Practices for Plugged Ducts"!

Are you tired of the discomfort and frustration that comes with plugged ducts disrupting your breastfeeding journey? Are you seeking gentle yet effective solutions to restore harmony and comfort to your body?

Look no further! This ebook is your comprehensive guide to reclaiming control over your breastfeeding experience and embracing the wellness you deserve.

In the pages that follow, you'll discover a treasure trove of natural remedies and self-care practices designed specifically for women who suffer from duct problems when breastfeeding, as well as those who want to prevent these challenges altogether.

 From soothing herbal compresses to gentle massage techniques, each strategy is meticulously crafted to alleviate discomfort and promote healing in a holistic and nurturing way.

But "From Discomfort to Relief" is more than just a guidebook—it's your roadmap to empowerment. As you dive into the chapters ahead, you'll not only learn practical solutions for a more comfortable and fulfilling breastfeeding experience but also cultivate a deeper understanding of your own body and its innate ability to heal.

So, dear reader, I invite you to embark on this journey of self-discovery and transformation with me. Together, let's unlock the power of natural remedies and self-care practices to bring comfort and relief to your life. Your breastfeeding journey is about to take a beautiful turn—let's dive in and discover the path to wellness together!

Chapter 1: Understanding Plugged Ducts:

Breastfeeding is a beautiful and natural way to nourish your baby, but it can also come with its challenges. One common issue that many breastfeeding mothers face is plugged ducts.

Plugged ducts can be painful and frustrating, but with the right knowledge and support, you can effectively manage and prevent them. In this comprehensive guide, we will explore what plugged ducts are, their causes, symptoms, treatment options, and prevention strategies.

What are Plugged Ducts?

Plugged ducts occur when one or more milk ducts in the breast become blocked, preventing the milk from flowing freely. This blockage can cause a build-up of milk behind the plug, leading to pain, swelling, and inflammation in the affected breast. Plugged ducts are a common issue for breastfeeding mothers, especially in the early weeks after giving birth.

Causes of Plugged Ducts

There are several factors that can contribute to the development of plugged ducts. Some common causes include:

- Inadequate milk removal: Plugged ducts often occur when

milk is not effectively removed from the breast. This can happen if your baby is not latching properly, if you are not breastfeeding or pumping frequently enough, or if there is a sudden change in your breastfeeding routine.

- Pressure on the breast: Wearing tight clothing, using a poorly fitting bra, or sleeping on your stomach can put pressure on the breast and contribute to the development of plugged ducts.

- Stress and fatigue: Stress and fatigue can weaken your immune system and make you more susceptible to developing plugged ducts. It is important to take care of yourself and prioritize rest and relaxation during the breastfeeding period.

- Engorgement: Engorgement occurs when your breasts become overly full of milk, leading to swelling and discomfort. This can increase the risk of developing plugged ducts.

Symptoms of Plugged Ducts

Plugged ducts can cause a variety of symptoms, including:

- Pain or tenderness in the affected breast
- Swelling and redness in the area of the plug
- A hard lump or knot in the breast
- Warmth or heat in the affected breast
- Decreased milk supply from the affected breast
- Flu-like symptoms, such as fever and chills

There are several treatment options available for plugged ducts, depending on the severity of the blockage. Some common treatment options include:

- Breastfeeding or pumping: Continuing to breastfeed or pump from the affected breast can help to clear the blockage and relieve the symptoms of plugged ducts. Make sure to position your baby properly and ensure a good latch to effectively remove the milk from the breast.

- Warm compress: Applying a warm compress to the affected breast can help to reduce pain and inflammation and promote milk flow. You can use a warm washcloth, a heating pad, or take a warm shower to help loosen the blockage.

- Massage: Gently massaging the affected breast can help to break up the plug and improve milk flow. You can massage the breast in a circular motion or use firm pressure to help release the blockage.

- Rest and hydration: Getting plenty of rest and staying hydrated can help to support your body's natural healing process and reduce the risk of developing plugged ducts.

- Over-the-counter pain relievers: If you are experiencing pain or discomfort from plugged ducts, you can take over-the-counter pain relievers, such as ibuprofen or acetaminophen, to help manage the symptoms.

If your symptoms do not improve with home remedies or if you develop a fever or other signs of infection, it is important to seek medical attention promptly. In some cases, antibiotics may be necessary to treat a severe or persistent plugged duct.

Prevention Strategies for Plugged Ducts

While plugged ducts can be a common occurrence for breastfeeding mothers, there are steps you can take to help prevent them from developing. Some effective prevention strategies include:

- Breastfeed frequently: Breastfeeding or pumping frequently helps to ensure that your breasts are emptied regularly and reduces the risk of developing plugged ducts. Aim to breastfeed every 2-3 hours during the day and at least once during the night.

- Ensure a good latch: Proper positioning and a good latch are essential for effective milk removal and can help prevent plugged ducts. Make sure your baby is latching correctly and seek help from a lactation consultant if you are experiencing difficulties.

- Avoid tight clothing: Wearing tight clothing or bras can put pressure on the breasts and contribute to the development of plugged ducts. Opt for loose-fitting, comfortable clothing that does not restrict the flow of milk.

The Science Behind Plugged Ducts and

Plugged ducts are a common issue that many breastfeeding mothers face. They occur when a milk duct in the breast becomes blocked, preventing milk from flowing freely. This can lead to pain, swelling, and even infection if not addressed promptly. Understanding the science behind plugged ducts can help mothers find relief and continue breastfeeding successfully.

The Science Behind Plugged Ducts

Plugged ducts can occur for a variety of reasons. One common cause is inadequate milk removal from the breast. This can happen if a baby is not latching properly, or if a mother is not emptying her breasts completely during feedings. When milk is not removed efficiently, it can build up in the ducts and lead to blockages.

Another common cause of plugged ducts is pressure on the breasts. This can happen if a mother wears tight- fitting bras or clothing, or if she sleeps on her stomach or with her breasts pressed against the mattress. Pressure on the breasts can compress the ducts and make it more difficult for milk to flow freely.

In some cases, plugged ducts can be caused by an overabundance of milk. When a mother produces more milk than her baby can consume, the breasts can become engorged and the ducts can become blocked. This is more common in the early weeks of breastfeeding when milk supply is still regulating.

Plugged ducts can also be caused by other factors such as stress, fatigue, dehydration, or illness. These factors can affect the immune system and make a mother more susceptible to developing plugged ducts.

Finding Relief from Plugged Ducts

If you are experiencing a plugged duct, there are several things you can do to find relief. The first step is to ensure that your baby is latching properly and emptying your breasts completely during feedings. This may require working with a lactation consultant to improve your baby's latch and feeding technique.

You can also try different breastfeeding positions to help drain your breasts more effectively. Experiment with different holds and angles to find the most comfortable and efficient position for you and your baby.

Applying heat to the affected breast can also help to relieve pain and swelling associated with plugged ducts. You can use a warm compress, a heating pad, or take a warm shower to help loosen the blockage and improve milk flow.

Massaging the affected breast can also help to break up the blockage and encourage milk to flow more freely. You can gently massage the breast in a circular motion, starting from the outer edges and working your way towards the nipple.

Frequent nursing or pumping can also help to clear a plugged duct. The more often you empty your breasts, the less likely you are to develop blockages. If your baby is not nursing effectively, you may need to pump after feedings to ensure that your breasts are fully drained.

If you are still experiencing pain and swelling after trying these remedies, you may need to consult with a healthcare provider. They can provide additional guidance and may recommend over-the-counter pain relievers

or prescription medications to help reduce inflammation and discomfort.

In some cases, a plugged duct can progress to a more serious condition called mastitis. Mastitis is an infection of the breast tissue that can cause flu-like symptoms such as fever, chills, and body aches. If you suspect that you have mastitis, it is important to seek medical attention promptly to prevent complications.

Preventing Plugged Ducts

While plugged ducts can be challenging to deal with, there are steps you can take to prevent them from occurring in the first place. One of the most important things you can do is to ensure that your baby is latching properly and nursing effectively. This will help to prevent milk from building up in the ducts and causing blockages.

You can also try to avoid pressure on the breasts by wearing loose-fitting clothing and bras, and by avoiding sleeping on your stomach or with your breasts pressed against the mattress. Taking breaks to rest and relax, staying hydrated, and eating a healthy diet can also help to reduce your risk of developing plugged ducts.

If you are prone to plugged ducts, you may benefit from using a breast pump to help drain your breasts more effectively. Pumping after feedings or during times when your baby is not nursing can help to prevent milk from building up in the ducts and causing blockages.

In conclusion, plugged ducts are a common issue that many breastfeeding mothers face. By understanding the science behind plugged ducts and taking proactive steps to prevent and treat them, you can find relief and continue breastfeeding successfully.

If you are experiencing persistent pain and swelling, it is important to seek medical attention to prevent complications such as mastitis. With the right support and guidance, you can overcome plugged ducts and enjoy a positive breastfeeding experience.

A Holistic Approach to Plugged Ducts From Discomfort to Relief

Breastfeeding is a beautiful and natural experience that provides numerous benefits for both mother and baby. However, it can also come with its fair share of challenges, one of the most common being plugged ducts.

Plugged ducts occur when milk flow is obstructed in the ducts of the breast, leading to pain, swelling, and discomfort for the breastfeeding mother.

While plugged ducts can be frustrating and painful, there are holistic approaches that can help alleviate the symptoms and promote healing. In this article, we will explore the causes of plugged ducts, the symptoms to look out for, and holistic remedies that can provide relief.

Causes of Plugged Ducts

Plugged ducts can be caused by a variety of factors, including:

- Poor milk drainage: Plugged ducts often occur when milk is not properly drained from the breast. This can happen if the baby does not latch correctly, if the mother is not breastfeeding frequently enough, or if there is an oversupply of milk.

- Pressure on the breast: Wearing tight-fitting bras or clothing, sleeping on your stomach, or carrying heavy bags can put pressure on the breasts and lead to plugged ducts.

- Stress: Stress can have a negative impact on milk production and flow, increasing the likelihood of plugged ducts.

- Hormonal changes: Fluctuations in hormone levels, such as those that occur during menstruation or weaning, can also contribute to plugged ducts.

Symptoms of Plugged Ducts

It is important to recognize the symptoms of plugged ducts so that you can address them promptly. Some common symptoms include:

- Pain or tenderness in the breast, often localized to a specific area
- Swelling or redness in the affected breast
- A hard lump or knot in the breast
- Warmth or heat in the affected area
- Fever or flu-like symptoms

If you are experiencing any of these symptoms, it is important to seek treatment as soon as possible to prevent the condition from worsening.

Holistic Remedies for Plugged Ducts

There are several holistic approaches that can help alleviate the symptoms of plugged ducts and promote healing.

Here are some effective remedies to consider:

1. Breastfeeding frequently: One of the best ways to prevent and treat plugged ducts is to breastfeed frequently and ensure that the breast is properly drained. Make sure that your baby is latching correctly and feeding on demand to help prevent milk from backing up in the ducts.

2. Warm compress: Applying a warm compress to the affected breast can help to reduce pain and swelling and promote milk flow. You can use a warm washcloth or a heating pad for this purpose.

3. Massage: Gently massaging the affected breast can help to break up the blockage and promote milk flow. You can do this while breastfeeding or pumping, using gentle circular motions towards the nipple.

4. Rest and relaxation: Stress can exacerbate plugged ducts, so it is important to take time to rest and relax. Practice deep breathing exercises, meditation, or yoga to help reduce stress levels and promote healing.

5. Hydration and nutrition: Staying hydrated and eating a healthy diet can help to support milk production and flow. Make sure to drink plenty of water and eat foods rich in vitamins and minerals, such as fruits, vegetables, and whole grains.

6. Herbal remedies: There are several herbal remedies that can help to alleviate the symptoms of plugged ducts. Fenugreek, blessed thistle, and alfalfa are all known for their lactation-promoting properties and can help to increase milk flow.

7. Essential oils: Certain essential oils, such as lavender, chamomile, and geranium, can help to reduce pain and inflammation associated with plugged ducts. Dilute a few drops of the essential oil in a carrier oil, such as coconut or olive oil, and massage into the affected breast.

8. Warm showers or baths: Taking a warm shower or bath can help to relax the muscles in the breast and promote milk flow. You can also try hand expressing in the shower to help clear the blockage.

9. Cold compress: In some cases, a cold compress can help to reduce swelling and inflammation in the affected breast. Apply a cold pack or a bag of frozen peas wrapped in a towel for 15-20 minutes at a time.

10. Chiropractic care: Some women find relief from plugged ducts through chiropractic adjustments. A chiropractor can help to realign the spine and promote proper nerve function, which can improve milk flow.

It is important to note that while these holistic remedies can be effective in treating plugged ducts, they are not a substitute for medical treatment. If you are experiencing severe pain, fever, or other concerning symptoms, it is important to seek advice from a healthcare provider.

Chapter 2: Natural Remedies for Plugged Ducts: Healing from Within

A plugged duct is a common issue that many breastfeeding mothers face. It occurs when a milk duct in the breast becomes blocked, causing milk to back up and create a painful lump. This can be a frustrating and uncomfortable experience, but there are natural remedies that can help to alleviate the symptoms and promote healing from within.

One of the most effective natural remedies for plugged ducts is frequent breastfeeding or pumping. By emptying the breast regularly, you can help to clear the blockage and prevent further build-up of milk.

It is important to make sure that your baby is latching properly and draining the breast completely during feedings. If you are exclusively pumping, be sure to empty both breasts fully during each session.

Another natural remedy for plugged ducts is heat therapy. Applying a warm compress to the affected breast can help to reduce inflammation and improve milk flow. You can use a warm washcloth, heating pad, or hot water bottle for this purpose. Take care not to make the compress too hot, as this can cause burns or damage to the skin. Heat therapy can be especially helpful before breastfeeding or pumping to help loosen the blockage and make it easier to clear.

Massage is another effective natural remedy for plugged ducts. Gently massaging the affected breast in a circular motion can help to break up the blockage and promote milk flow.

You can do this while in the shower or bath, or before or after breastfeeding or pumping. Be sure to use gentle pressure and avoid pressing too hard, as this can cause further discomfort or damage to the breast tissue.

In addition to heat therapy and massage, there are several herbal remedies that can help to alleviate the symptoms of plugged ducts.

One popular option is lecithin, a supplement that can help to reduce the stickiness of breast milk and prevent blockages from forming. You can find lecithin in capsule form at most health food stores, and it is generally safe for breastfeeding mothers to take.

Another herbal remedy for plugged ducts is fenugreek. This herb is known for its ability to increase milk supply and promote healthy breastfeeding.

You can take fenugreek supplements or drink fenugreek tea to help clear blocked ducts and prevent future issues. Be sure to consult with a healthcare provider before taking any herbal remedies, especially if you are pregnant or nursing.

In addition to these natural remedies, there are several lifestyle changes that can help to prevent plugged ducts from occurring. It is important to stay well-hydrated and eat a balanced diet rich in fruits, vegetables, and whole grains.

Avoid wearing tight clothing or bras that can constrict the breasts and impede milk flow. Make sure to get plenty of rest and avoid stress, as these factors can contribute to blocked ducts.

If you are experiencing persistent or severe symptoms of plugged ducts, it is important to seek medical attention. A healthcare provider can help to diagnose the issue and recommend appropriate treatment options.

In some cases, a plugged duct may lead to mastitis, a more serious infection of the breast tissue that requires antibiotics to treat. It is important to address any issues with breastfeeding or milk supply as soon as possible to prevent complications and promote healing.

In conclusion, plugged ducts are a common issue that many breastfeeding mothers face, but there are natural remedies that can help to alleviate the symptoms and promote healing from within. By using frequent breastfeeding or pumping, heat therapy, massage, and herbal remedies, you can help to clear blocked ducts and prevent future issues. It is important to make healthy lifestyle choices and seek medical attention if needed to ensure a successful breastfeeding experience. With the right care and support, you can overcome plugged ducts and continue to provide your baby with the nourishment they need.

Self-Care Practices for Plugged Ducts: Nurturing Your Body

Self-care practices are essential for maintaining overall health and well-being. When it comes to plugged ducts, self-care becomes even more important to prevent further complications and promote healing.

Plugged ducts can occur when milk is not effectively removed from the breast, leading to a blockage in the milk duct. This can cause pain, swelling, and inflammation in the affected breast, making breastfeeding uncomfortable and potentially leading to more serious issues such as mastitis.

In order to effectively manage plugged ducts, it is important to incorporate self-care practices into your daily routine. By nurturing your body and taking steps to promote healing, you can alleviate symptoms, prevent further blockages, and continue breastfeeding successfully.

In this article, we will explore some self-care practices for plugged ducts that can help you nurture your body and support your breastfeeding journey.

1. Breastfeed frequently and effectively

One of the best ways to prevent and manage plugged ducts is to breastfeed frequently and effectively. Make sure your baby is latching correctly and breastfeeding on demand to ensure that milk is being effectively removed from the breast.

If you are experiencing pain or discomfort while breastfeeding, seek support from a lactation consultant or healthcare provider to address any issues that may be contributing to plugged ducts.

2. Apply heat

Applying heat to the affected breast can help to relieve pain and inflammation associated with plugged ducts. You can use a warm compress, heating pad, or take a warm shower to help open up the milk duct and promote milk flow.

Heat can also help to relax the muscles in the breast and reduce swelling, making breastfeeding more comfortable.

3. Massage the affected breast

Gentle massage can help to break up the blockage in the milk duct and promote milk flow. You can use your fingers or a warm washcloth to massage the affected breast in a circular motion, moving towards the nipple. This can help to release the trapped milk and alleviate pain and discomfort associated with plugged ducts.

4. Practice good hygiene

Maintaining good hygiene is important when managing plugged ducts to prevent infection and promote healing. Make sure to wash your hands before breastfeeding or pumping to prevent the spread of bacteria.

You can also use a warm washcloth to gently cleanse the affected breast before and after breastfeeding to keep the area clean and prevent further blockages.

5. Stay hydrated

Staying hydrated is essential for maintaining a healthy milk supply and preventing plugged ducts. Make sure to drink plenty of water throughout the day to keep your body hydrated and support milk production. Dehydration can lead to thicker, more concentrated milk that is more likely to cause blockages in the milk ducts.

6. Get plenty of rest

Rest is crucial for promoting healing and preventing further complications from plugged ducts. Make sure to prioritize rest and relaxation, especially if you are experiencing pain or discomfort. Take breaks throughout the day to rest and recover, and consider asking for help with household tasks or childcare to give yourself the time and space you need to heal.

7. Use a breast pump

If you are having difficulty breastfeeding due to plugged ducts, you can use a breast pump to help remove milk from the affected breast. Pumping can help to relieve engorgement and prevent further blockages in the milk ducts. Make sure to use the correct size flange and follow the manufacturer's instructions for proper use of the breast pump.

8. Wear loose, comfortable clothing

Tight clothing can restrict milk flow and contribute to plugged ducts. Opt for loose, comfortable clothing that does not constrict the breasts to promote healthy milk flow and prevent blockages.

Consider wearing a supportive bra that provides gentle compression without being too tight to help alleviate pain and discomfort associated with plugged ducts.

9. Apply cold packs

In addition to heat, cold packs can also help to reduce pain and inflammation associated with plugged ducts. You can use a cold pack or ice pack wrapped in a towel to apply gentle pressure to the affected breast and help reduce swelling. Cold packs can also help to numb the area and provide relief from discomfort.

10. Seek support

Managing plugged ducts can be challenging, both physically and emotionally. It is important to seek support from a healthcare provider, lactation consultant, or support group to help you navigate this difficult time.
Talking to other breastfeeding mothers who have experienced plugged ducts can provide valuable insight and support as you

work to overcome this common breastfeeding issue.

In conclusion, self-care practices are essential for managing plugged ducts and promoting healing in the affected breast. By incorporating these self-care practices into your daily routine, you can nurture your body, alleviate symptoms, and prevent further complications from plugged ducts.

Remember to prioritize rest, hydration, and effective breastfeeding techniques to support your breastfeeding journey and maintain overall health and well- being. If you are experiencing persistent pain, swelling, or inflammation in the breast, seek support from a healthcare provider to address any underlying issues and ensure that you are on the path to healing.

Chapter: The Importance of Early Detection and Treatment for Plugged Ducts

Plugged ducts are a common issue that many breastfeeding mothers face. It occurs when milk flow is blocked in the milk ducts, leading to pain, swelling, and potentially serious complications if left untreated.

Early detection and treatment of plugged ducts are crucial in preventing further discomfort and ensuring successful breastfeeding. In this article, we will discuss the importance of early detection and treatment for plugged ducts in breastfeeding mothers.

Breastfeeding is a natural and beneficial way to nourish your baby, but it can also come with its own set of challenges. Plugged ducts are one of the most common issues that breastfeeding mothers encounter.

They can occur for a variety of reasons, such as improper latching, infrequent feedings, or even tight clothing that puts pressure on the breasts. When a milk duct becomes blocked, it can lead to a build-up of milk, inflammation, and pain in the affected breast.

Early detection of plugged ducts is crucial in preventing further complications. One of the first signs of a plugged duct is a localized area of tenderness or pain in the breast. This discomfort may be accompanied by swelling, redness, and a feeling of fullness in the affected breast. Some women may also experience a low-grade fever or flu-like symptoms when they have a plugged duct.

If you suspect that you have a plugged duct, it is important to take action immediately. Ignoring the symptoms and hoping that they will go away on their own can lead to more serious complications, such as mastitis or abscess formation.

Early detection and treatment of plugged ducts can help to alleviate pain and discomfort, prevent infection, and ensure that breastfeeding can continue successfully.

There are several steps that you can take to help clear a plugged duct and prevent further complications. One of the most effective ways to treat a plugged duct is to nurse frequently on the affected breast.

The suction from your baby's mouth can help to loosen the blockage and promote milk flow. You can also try massaging the affected breast while nursing or applying warm compresses to help relieve pain and swelling.

In addition to nursing frequently, it is important to ensure that you are using proper breastfeeding techniques to prevent plugged ducts from occurring in the first place. Make sure that your baby is latching correctly and emptying the breast fully during feedings. Avoid wearing tight clothing or bras that can put pressure on the breasts and restrict milk flow. If you are experiencing frequent plugged ducts, consider consulting with a lactation consultant for additional support and guidance.

If you are unable to clear a plugged duct on your own or if you are experiencing severe pain or other concerning symptoms, it is important to seek medical attention.

Your healthcare provider may recommend using a breast pump to help empty the affected breast more effectively or prescribe medication to help reduce inflammation and pain. In some cases, a healthcare provider may need to manually remove the blockage or perform a procedure to drain any accumulated fluid.

Early detection and treatment of plugged ducts are essential in ensuring that breastfeeding can continue successfully and that both mother and baby remain healthy. By taking proactive steps to address plugged ducts as soon as they occur, you can prevent further discomfort and complications and promote a positive breastfeeding experience for both you and your baby.

In conclusion, plugged ducts are a common issue that many breastfeeding mothers face, but early detection and treatment are key in preventing further complications.

By recognizing the signs of a plugged duct and taking prompt action to address it, you can alleviate pain and discomfort, prevent infection, and ensure that breastfeeding can continue successfully. If you are experiencing symptoms of a plugged duct, do not hesitate to seek help from a healthcare provider or lactation consultant.

Chapter 3: Breaking the Cycle: Preventing Plugged Ducts Before They Happen

Breastfeeding is a beautiful and natural way for mothers to nourish their babies. However, it can also come with its own set of challenges, one of which is plugged ducts. Plugged ducts occur when milk flow is blocked in a milk duct, leading to pain, swelling, and potential infection.

This can be a frustrating and uncomfortable experience for breastfeeding mothers, but the good news is that there are steps you can take to prevent plugged ducts before they happen.

In this article, we will discuss the causes of plugged ducts, the symptoms to watch out for, and most importantly, how to prevent them from occurring in the first place. By following these preventive measures, you can help ensure a smooth and comfortable breastfeeding experience for both you and your baby.

Causes of Plugged Ducts

Plugged ducts can be caused by a variety of factors, but the most common culprits include:

1. Poor Latch: A poor latch can prevent your baby from

effectively draining your breast, leading to milk build- up and potential blockages in the ducts.

2. Infrequent Feedings: Infrequent feedings can also contribute to plugged ducts, as milk can accumulate in the ducts when not regularly emptied.

3. Tight Clothing: Wearing tight-fitting bras or clothing can put pressure on the breasts, potentially causing milk flow to become blocked.

4. Stress: Stress can have a negative impact on milk production and flow, increasing the likelihood of plugged ducts.

5. Fatigue: Lack of sleep and exhaustion can also affect milk flow and increase the risk of plugged ducts.

Symptoms of Plugged Ducts

It's important to be aware of the symptoms of plugged ducts so that you can address them promptly. Common symptoms include:

1. Pain or tenderness in the breast, often localized to one area
2. Swelling or redness in the affected area
3. A lump or firmness in the breast
4. Warmth or heat coming from the affected area
5. Fever or flu-like symptoms

If you are experiencing any of these symptoms, it's important to seek help from a lactation consultant or healthcare provider to prevent further complications such as mastitis, a more serious breast infection.

Preventing Plugged Ducts Before They Happen

Now that we've discussed the causes and symptoms of plugged ducts, let's explore some preventive measures you
can take to avoid this uncomfortable condition:

1. Ensure a Good Latch: A proper latch is essential for effective breastfeeding. Make sure your baby is latching onto your breast correctly to ensure that milk is being efficiently drained from the breast.

2. Feed Frequently: Aim to breastfeed your baby every 2-3 hours or whenever they show signs of hunger. Regular feedings help prevent milk build-up and keep the ducts clear.

3. Empty the Breast Completely: Make sure your baby is draining each breast fully during feedings. If your baby doesn't empty one breast completely, offer the same breast again before switching to the other side.

4. Use Different Breastfeeding Positions: Changing up your breastfeeding positions can help ensure that all parts of the breast are being emptied properly. Experiment with different positions to find what works best for you and your baby.

5. Avoid Tight Clothing: Opt for loose-fitting bras and clothing

that won't constrict your breasts. This will help prevent pressure on the ducts and promote healthy milk flow.

6. Manage Stress: Finding ways to reduce stress and relax can help maintain a healthy milk supply and prevent plugged ducts. Practice deep breathing, meditation, or other relaxation techniques to help manage stress.

7. Get Adequate Rest: Make sure you are getting enough rest and sleep to support your body's milk production. Listen to your body and prioritize self-care to prevent fatigue and exhaustion.

8. Stay Hydrated: Drinking plenty of water is essential for breastfeeding mothers. Stay hydrated to support milk production and prevent dehydration, which can contribute to plugged ducts.

9. Massage Your Breasts: Gentle breast massage can help promote milk flow and prevent blockages in the ducts. Try massaging your breasts in a circular motion before and after feedings.

10. Apply Heat: Applying a warm compress to the affected breast can help relieve pain and encourage milk flow. Use a warm washcloth or a heating pad for 10-15 minutes before feedings.

11. Nurse on Demand: Respond to your baby's hunger cues and nurse on demand. This will help prevent milk build-up and keep the ducts clear.

12. Avoid Abrupt Weaning: Gradually wean your baby from breastfeeding to prevent sudden changes in milk supply, which can lead to plugged ducts. Consult a lactation consultant for guidance on gentle weaning methods.

By following these preventive measures, you can reduce the risk of plugged ducts and enjoy a more comfortable breastfeeding experience.

Overcoming Obstacles: Strategies for Clearing Plugged Ducts

Breastfeeding is a beautiful and natural process that provides numerous benefits for both mother and baby. However, it can also come with its fair share of challenges, one of which is plugged ducts. Plugged ducts occur when milk flow is blocked in a milk duct, causing pain, swelling, and discomfort for the breastfeeding mother.

This can be a frustrating and painful experience, but there are strategies and techniques that can help clear plugged ducts and alleviate symptoms.

In this article, we will discuss the causes of plugged ducts, the symptoms to look out for, and effective strategies for clearing them.

We will also provide tips for preventing plugged ducts in the future. By understanding how to overcome this common breastfeeding obstacle, mothers can continue to breastfeed successfully and comfortably.

Causes of Plugged Ducts

Plugged ducts can occur for a variety of reasons, but they are most commonly caused by a build-up of milk in a milk duct. This can happen if milk is not effectively removed from the breast, leading to a blockage in the duct. Some common causes of plugged ducts include:

- Infrequent or incomplete breastfeeding or pumping sessions: If a mother does not breastfeed or pump regularly, milk can build up in the breast and cause a blockage in the duct.

- Pressure on the breast: Wearing tight-fitting bras or clothing, sleeping on the stomach, or carrying heavy bags on the shoulder can put pressure on the breast and lead to plugged ducts.

- Poor latch: A poor latch can prevent the baby from effectively removing milk from the breast, leading to a build-up of milk in the duct.

- Stress or fatigue: Stress and fatigue can impact milk production and flow, making it more likely for plugged ducts to occur.
- Mastitis: Plugged ducts can sometimes be a precursor to mastitis, an infection of the breast tissue that can cause fever, chills, and flu-like symptoms.

Symptoms of Plugged Ducts

It is important for breastfeeding mothers to be aware of the symptoms of plugged ducts so that they can take action to clear them as soon as possible. Some common symptoms of plugged ducts include:

- Pain or tenderness in the breast, often in a specific area
- Swelling or redness in the affected area

- A hard lump or knot in the breast
- Warmth or heat in the affected area
- Discomfort or pain while breastfeeding
- Decreased milk supply from the affected breast

If you are experiencing any of these symptoms, it is important to take steps to clear the plugged duct as soon as possible to prevent further complications.

Strategies for Clearing Plugged Ducts

There are several strategies and techniques that can help clear plugged ducts and alleviate symptoms. It is

important to continue breastfeeding or pumping from the affected breast to help remove the blockage and prevent further complications. Here are some effective strategies for clearing plugged ducts:

1. Massage: Gentle massage of the affected breast can help to break up the blockage and promote milk flow. Use circular motions and gentle pressure to massage the affected area while breastfeeding or pumping.

2. Warm compress: Applying a warm compress to the affected breast can help to reduce pain and swelling and promote milk flow. Use a warm washcloth or heating pad on the affected area for 10-15 minutes before breastfeeding or pumping.

3. Hot shower: Taking a hot shower can help to relax the muscles in the breast and promote milk flow. Stand under the

hot water and gently massage the affected breast to help clear the blockage.

4. Nurse frequently: Breastfeeding or pumping frequently can help to keep milk flowing and prevent blockages from forming. Try to breastfeed on demand or pump every 2-3 hours to help clear the plugged duct.

5. Change positions: Changing breastfeeding positions can help to ensure that all areas of the breast are being emptied effectively. Experiment with different positions, such as the football hold or side-lying position, to help clear the blockage.

6. Use a breast pump: If breastfeeding alone is not effective in clearing the plugged duct, using a breast pump can help to empty the breast more thoroughly. Pumping after breastfeeding can help to remove any remaining milk and clear the blockage.

7. Stay hydrated: Drinking plenty of water can help to keep milk flowing and prevent blockages from forming. Aim to drink at least 8-10 glasses of water per day to stay hydrated and support milk production.

8. Rest and relax: Stress and fatigue can impact milk production and flow, making it more likely for plugged ducts to occur. Take time to rest and relax, practice deep breathing exercises, and prioritize self-care to help clear the blockage.
Over-the-counter remedies: Some over-the-counter remedies, such as lecithin supplements or ibuprofen, can help to reduce pain and inflammation associated with plugged ducts.

Finding Balance: Managing Plugged Ducts with a Busy Lifestyle

Finding balance between managing plugged ducts and a busy lifestyle can be a challenging task for many breastfeeding mothers. Plugged ducts are a common issue that can occur when milk ducts become blocked, causing discomfort and potentially leading to more serious issues like mastitis.

This can be especially difficult to navigate when trying to juggle the demands of work, family, and other responsibilities. However, with some strategic planning and self-care practices, it is possible to find a balance that allows for effective management of plugged ducts while still maintaining a busy lifestyle.

One of the first steps in finding balance is understanding the causes and symptoms of plugged ducts. Plugged ducts can occur for a variety of reasons, including inadequate milk removal, pressure on the breast from tight clothing or a poorly fitting bra, and even stress.

Symptoms of plugged ducts can include a tender or painful lump in the breast, redness or warmth in the affected area, and a decrease in milk supply. By being aware of these potential causes and symptoms, breastfeeding mothers can take proactive steps to prevent and manage plugged ducts before they become a more serious issue.

One key aspect of managing plugged ducts with a busy lifestyle is ensuring that breastfeeding mothers have the time and space to properly empty their breasts.

This may require finding moments throughout the day to pump or nurse, even when juggling other responsibilities. Setting aside dedicated time for breastfeeding or pumping can help ensure that milk is being effectively removed from the breasts, reducing the risk of developing plugged ducts.

Additionally, finding a comfortable and private space to nurse or pump can help reduce stress and allow for a more relaxed breastfeeding experience.

In addition to finding time for breastfeeding or pumping, it is important for breastfeeding mothers to prioritize self-care practices that can help prevent and manage plugged ducts. This can include staying hydrated, eating a balanced diet, getting enough rest, and managing stress levels.

Engaging in regular physical activity can also help promote healthy milk flow and prevent blocked ducts. By taking care of their own physical and emotional well- being, breastfeeding mothers can better manage the demands of a busy lifestyle while still prioritizing their breastfeeding goals.

It can also be helpful for breastfeeding mothers to seek support from healthcare professionals, lactation consultants, and other breastfeeding mothers who have experience managing plugged ducts.

These individuals can provide valuable advice, guidance, and encouragement to help breastfeeding mothers navigate the challenges of plugged ducts while balancing a busy lifestyle.

Seeking support from others who understand the unique challenges of breastfeeding can help alleviate feelings of isolation and provide reassurance that breastfeeding mothers are not alone in their struggles.

In some cases, managing plugged ducts may require more intensive interventions, such as using warm compresses, massaging the affected area, or taking over-the-counter pain relievers.

If plugged ducts persist or worsen, it is important for breastfeeding mothers to seek medical attention from a healthcare provider. In some cases, a healthcare provider may recommend antibiotics to treat an infection or other interventions to help resolve the issue.

By being proactive about seeking medical attention when needed, breastfeeding mothers can ensure that plugged ducts are effectively managed and do not interfere with their busy lifestyle.

Finding balance between managing plugged ducts and a busy lifestyle is a process that requires patience, perseverance, and self-care. By prioritizing breastfeeding goals, seeking support from healthcare professionals and other breastfeeding mothers, and taking proactive steps to prevent and manage plugged ducts, breastfeeding mothers can successfully navigate the challenges of breastfeeding while still maintaining a busy lifestyle.

With the right strategies and support systems in place, breastfeeding mothers can find a balance that allows for effective management of plugged ducts while still meeting the demands of work, family, and other responsibilities.

Chapter 4: Healing Hands: Massage Techniques for Plugged Ducts

Breastfeeding is a beautiful and natural process that provides numerous benefits for both mother and baby. However, it is not without its challenges. One common issue that many breastfeeding mothers face is plugged ducts. Plugged ducts can be painful and uncomfortable, but there are ways to help alleviate the symptoms and promote healing.

Massage techniques can be incredibly beneficial for treating plugged ducts. By using gentle and targeted massage techniques, you can help to break up the blockage in the duct and promote the flow of milk. In this article, we will explore some effective massage techniques for treating plugged ducts and promoting healing.

What are Plugged Ducts?

Plugged ducts occur when a milk duct in the breast becomes blocked, preventing the flow of milk. This blockage can be caused by a variety of factors, including inadequate milk removal, pressure on the breast, or a change in feeding patterns.

Plugged ducts are often characterized by a tender lump in the breast, redness, and pain. If left untreated, plugged ducts can lead to more serious issues, such as mastitis.

Massage Techniques for Plugged Ducts

Massage can be a highly effective way to help treat plugged ducts. By using gentle and targeted massage techniques, you can help to break up the blockage in the duct and promote the flow of milk. Here are some massage techniques that can help to alleviate the symptoms of plugged ducts and promote healing:

1. Warm Compress: Before beginning any massage techniques, it can be helpful to apply a warm compress to the affected breast. The heat from the compress can help to relax the muscles and ducts in the breast, making it easier to massage out the blockage.

2. Circular Massage: To perform a circular massage, use your fingertips to gently massage the affected area in a circular motion. Start at the outer edge of the breast and work your way towards the nipple. This can help to break up the blockage and promote the flow of milk.

3. Lymphatic Drainage Massage: Lymphatic drainage massage is a gentle massage technique that can help to reduce swelling and promote lymphatic flow. To perform lymphatic drainage massage, use gentle pressure to massage the affected breast in a downward motion towards the armpit. This can help to reduce inflammation and promote healing.

4. Reverse Pressure Softening: Reverse pressure softening is a

technique that can help to soften the blockage in the duct and make it easier to massage out. To perform reverse pressure softening, use your fingertips to gently apply pressure around the lump in a circular motion. This can help to break up the blockage and promote the flow of milk.

5. Hand Expression: In addition to massage techniques, hand expression can also be helpful for treating plugged ducts. Hand expression involves using your hand to manually express milk from the affected breast. This can help to relieve pressure on the duct and promote the flow of milk.

6. Breast Compression: Breast compression is another technique that can help to promote the flow of milk and

alleviate the symptoms of plugged ducts. To perform breast compression, use your hand to gently compress the breast while your baby is nursing. This can help to ensure that the milk is fully emptied from the breast and prevent further blockages.

7. Self-Massage: Self-massage can be a convenient and effective way to treat plugged ducts. To perform self- massage, use your fingertips to gently massage the affected breast in a circular motion. You can also use a massage tool, such as a massage ball or roller, to help break up the blockage and promote healing.

8. Warm Shower: Taking a warm shower can also be beneficial for treating plugged ducts. The heat from the shower can help to relax the muscles and ducts in the breast, making it easier to massage out the blockage. You can also use a handheld

massager or showerhead to target specific areas of the breast.

9. Cool Compress: After performing massage techniques, it can be helpful to apply a cool compress to the affected breast. The cool temperature can help to reduce inflammation and provide relief from pain and discomfort.

10. Consult a Lactation Consultant: If you are experiencing persistent plugged ducts, it may be helpful to consult a lactation consultant. A lactation consultant can provide personalized guidance and support to help you effectively treat plugged ducts and prevent future blockages.

In addition to these massage techniques, it is important to ensure that you are properly emptying your breasts during feedings. Make sure that your baby is latching correctly and nursing effectively. You can also try different breastfeeding positions to help ensure that your breasts are fully emptied.

Preventing Plugged Ducts

While massage techniques can be effective for treating plugged ducts, it is also important to take steps to prevent them from occurring in the first place.

Soothing Solutions: Herbal Remedies for Plugged Ducts Soothing Solutions

Breastfeeding is a beautiful and natural way to nourish your baby, but it can come with its challenges. One common issue that many breastfeeding mothers face is plugged ducts.

A plugged duct occurs when a milk duct in the breast becomes blocked, causing milk to back up and create a painful lump. This can be a frustrating and uncomfortable experience for any breastfeeding mother, but there are natural remedies that can help alleviate the discomfort and clear the blockage.

Herbal remedies have been used for centuries to treat a variety of ailments, including plugged ducts. These natural solutions can help reduce inflammation, improve milk flow, and relieve pain associated with plugged ducts. In this article, we will explore some of the most effective herbal remedies for plugged ducts and how they can help you find relief.

1. Echinacea

Echinacea is a powerful herb that is known for its immune-boosting properties. It can help reduce inflammation and fight off infection, making it an excellent remedy for plugged ducts. Echinacea can be taken in supplement form or brewed into a tea to help support your immune system and promote healing. It is important to consult with a healthcare provider before using echinacea, especially if you have any underlying health conditions or are taking medications.

2. Dandelion

Dandelion is another herbal remedy that can be beneficial for treating plugged ducts. It is a natural diuretic, which means it can help reduce fluid retention and swelling in the breast. Dandelion can be brewed into a tea or taken in supplement form to help improve milk flow and clear blockages in the milk ducts. It is important to stay hydrated while using dandelion to help support the body's natural detoxification process.

3. Fenugreek

Fenugreek is a popular herb that is commonly used to help increase milk supply in breastfeeding mothers. It can also be effective in treating plugged ducts by promoting milk flow and reducing inflammation in the breast.

Fenugreek can be taken in supplement form or brewed into a tea to help relieve pain and discomfort associated with plugged ducts. It is important to consult with a lactation consultant or healthcare provider before using fenugreek, especially if you have a history of allergies or are taking medications.

4. Marshmallow Root

Marshmallow root is a soothing herb that can help reduce inflammation and promote healing in the breast tissue. It can be brewed into a tea or applied topically as a poultice to help relieve pain and discomfort associated with plugged ducts.

Marshmallow root can also help improve milk flow and clear blockages in the milk ducts. It is important to consult with a healthcare provider before using marshmallow root, especially if you have any underlying health conditions or are taking medications.

5. Red Clover

Red clover is a gentle herb that is known for its hormone-balancing properties. It can help regulate estrogen levels in the body, which can be beneficial for breastfeeding mothers experiencing plugged ducts. Red clover can be brewed into a tea or taken in supplement form to help reduce inflammation and improve milk flow. It is important to consult with a healthcare provider before using red clover, especially if you have a history of hormone-related conditions or are taking medications.

6. Thyme

Thyme is a fragrant herb that is commonly used in cooking, but it also has medicinal properties that can be beneficial for treating plugged ducts. Thyme is a natural antimicrobial and can help fight off infection in the breast tissue. It can be brewed into a tea or applied topically as a poultice to help reduce inflammation and promote healing. Thyme can also help improve milk flow and clear blockages in the milk ducts. It is important to consult with a healthcare provider before using thyme, especially if you have any underlying health conditions or are taking medications.

7. Sage

Sage is an herb that is known for its drying properties, which can be beneficial for treating plugged ducts. It can help reduce milk production and alleviate engorgement in the breast.

Sage can be brewed into a tea or applied topically as a poultice to help relieve pain and discomfort associated with plugged ducts. It is important to consult with a healthcare provider before using sage, especially if you have a history of hormone-related conditions or are taking medications.

8. Chamomile

Chamomile is a calming herb that can help reduce stress and promote relaxation in breastfeeding mothers. It can also be effective in treating plugged ducts by reducing inflammation and improving milk flow.

Chamomile can be brewed into a tea or applied topically as a poultice to help relieve pain and discomfort associated with plugged ducts.

The Power of Heat Therapy for Plugged Duct Relief

Heat therapy is a popular and effective method for relieving plugged ducts in breastfeeding mothers. Plugged ducts occur when milk is not effectively removed from the breast, leading to a blockage in the milk duct.

 This can be a painful and frustrating experience for many breastfeeding mothers, but heat therapy can help to alleviate the discomfort and help to clear the blockage.

Heat therapy works by increasing blood flow to the affected area, which can help to reduce inflammation and improve the flow of milk through the duct.

This can help to loosen the blockage and make it easier for the milk to flow freely. Heat therapy can also help to relax the muscles around the duct, making it easier for the milk to pass through.

There are several ways that heat therapy can be used to relieve plugged ducts. One common method is to apply a warm compress to the affected breast.

This can be done by soaking a cloth in warm water and placing it on the breast for 10-15 minutes. The heat from the compress can help to increase blood flow and reduce inflammation in the duct, making it easier for the milk to flow.

Another popular method of heat therapy for plugged ducts is to take a warm shower or bath. The heat from the water can help to relax the muscles around the duct and improve the flow of milk. Some mothers find that massaging the affected breast while in the shower can also help to clear the blockage and relieve the pain.

In addition to warm compresses and showers, some mothers find relief from plugged ducts by using a heating pad or hot water bottle on the affected breast.

This can provide a consistent source of heat to the area, helping to reduce inflammation and improve milk flow. It is important to use caution when using a heating pad or hot water bottle, as excessive heat can damage the skin and cause burns.

In addition to heat therapy, there are several other methods that can help to relieve plugged ducts in breastfeeding mothers. Massaging the affected breast can help to loosen the blockage and improve milk flow.

Some mothers find that changing breastfeeding positions can also help to clear the duct and relieve the pain. It is important to continue breastfeeding regularly, as this can help to prevent future blockages from occurring.

If heat therapy and other home remedies do not provide relief, it is important to seek help from a healthcare provider. A lactation consultant or healthcare provider can provide additional support and guidance on how to effectively treat plugged ducts.

In some cases, a healthcare provider may recommend medications or other treatments to help clear the blockage and relieve the pain.

Overall, heat therapy is a powerful and effective method for relieving plugged ducts in breastfeeding mothers. By increasing blood flow to the affected area and relaxing the muscles around the duct, heat therapy can help to clear the blockage and improve milk flow.

It is important to use caution when using heat therapy, and to seek help from a healthcare provider if home remedies do not provide relief.

With the right treatment and support, plugged ducts can be effectively treated, allowing breastfeeding mothers to continue to provide their babies with the important benefits of breast milk.

Chapter 5: Cultivating Inner Peace Mindful Practices for Plugged

Breastfeeding is a beautiful and natural way to nourish your baby, but it can also come with its challenges. One common issue that breastfeeding mothers may face is plugged ducts.

A plugged duct occurs when a milk duct becomes blocked, causing milk to back up and create a painful lump in the breast.

This can be a frustrating and uncomfortable experience for many mothers, but there are mindful practices that can help alleviate the symptoms and promote healing.

In this article, we will explore some mindful practices that breastfeeding mothers can incorporate into their routine to help prevent and treat plugged ducts. By cultivating inner peace and practicing self-care, mothers can navigate the challenges of breastfeeding with grace and resilience.

Mindfulness and Breastfeeding

Mindfulness is the practice of being present in the moment and fully engaging with your thoughts, feelings, and sensations. When it comes to breastfeeding, mindfulness can be a powerful tool for promoting relaxation, reducing stress, and enhancing the bonding experience between mother and baby.

When a mother is mindful during breastfeeding, she is better able to tune into her body's signals and respond to her baby's needs.

This can help prevent issues like plugged ducts, as the mother is more attuned to her body's cues and can take proactive steps to address any discomfort or tension.

Incorporating mindfulness into your breastfeeding routine can be as simple as taking a few deep breaths before each feeding, closing your eyes and focusing on the sensations of breastfeeding, or practicing gentle stretches or relaxation techniques while nursing.

By bringing mindfulness into your breastfeeding practice, you can create a sense of calm and peace that can help prevent plugged ducts and promote overall well-being.

Preventing Plugged Ducts with Mindful Practices

While plugged ducts can occur for a variety of reasons, there are some mindful practices that breastfeeding mothers can incorporate into their routine to help prevent this common issue.

By taking proactive steps to care for your body and mind, you can reduce your risk of developing plugged ducts and promote a healthy breastfeeding experience for both you and your baby.

1. Stay Hydrated: One of the most important ways to prevent

plugged ducts is to stay hydrated. Drinking plenty of water throughout the day can help keep your milk flowing smoothly and prevent blockages in the milk ducts.

2.   Make a conscious effort to drink water regularly, especially before and after breastfeeding sessions, to support your body's natural processes and prevent plugged ducts from occurring.

3. Practice Gentle Breast Massage: Gentle breast massage can help promote circulation in the breast tissue and prevent blockages in the milk ducts.

4. Before or after breastfeeding, take a few moments to gently massage your breasts in a circular motion, starting at the outer edges and working your way towards the nipple. This can help release any tension or tightness in the breast tissue and prevent plugged ducts from forming.

5. Use Warm Compresses: Applying a warm compress to the affected breast can help promote milk flow and

reduce inflammation in the milk ducts. Before breastfeeding or pumping, place a warm washcloth or heating pad on the affected breast for a few minutes to help soften the breast tissue and encourage milk to flow more freely. This can help prevent plugged ducts and alleviate any discomfort or pain associated with this common issue.

6. Practice Relaxation Techniques: Stress and tension can contribute to the development of plugged ducts, so it's important to practice relaxation techniques to help promote a sense of

calm and peace during breastfeeding. Before each feeding, take a few deep breaths, close your eyes, and focus on the sensations of breastfeeding. This can help relax your body and mind, reduce stress, and promote a healthy breastfeeding experience for both you and your baby.

7. Maintain Good Breastfeeding Posture: Proper breastfeeding posture is essential for preventing plugged ducts and promoting healthy milk flow.

When breastfeeding, make sure to sit upright with your back supported and your baby positioned at the breast in a way that allows for optimal milk transfer.

Avoid slouching or leaning forward, as this can put pressure on the milk ducts and increase your risk of developing plugged ducts. By maintaining good breastfeeding posture, you can help prevent plugged ducts and promote a comfortable and effective breastfeeding experience.

Treating Plugged Ducts with Mindful Practices

Despite your best efforts to prevent plugged ducts, it's possible that you may still experience this common issue at some point during your breastfeeding journey. If you develop a plugged duct, there are mindful practices that you can incorporate into your routine to help alleviate the symptoms and promote healing.

Nurse Frequently: One of the most effective ways to treat a

plugged duct is to nurse frequently and empty the affected breast completely. Breastfeeding or pumping more often can help promote milk flow and reduce the blockage in the milk duct.

Nutrition and Plugged Ducts: Fueling Your Body for Healing

Nutrition plays a crucial role in the healing process, especially when it comes to plugged ducts. Plugged ducts can occur in breastfeeding mothers when milk flow is obstructed, leading to pain, swelling, and potential infection.

 Proper nutrition can help support the body's healing process and prevent future plugged ducts from occurring. In this article, we will explore the importance of nutrition in healing plugged ducts and provide some dietary recommendations to help fuel your body for recovery.

Plugged ducts are a common issue that many breastfeeding mothers face. They can be caused by a variety of factors, including poor latch, infrequent feedings, tight clothing, and stress.

When a duct becomes blocked, milk can back up and cause inflammation, pain, and swelling in the affected breast. If left untreated, a plugged duct can lead to mastitis, a more serious infection that requires medical intervention.

One of the key ways to prevent and treat plugged ducts is through proper nutrition. A well-balanced diet can help support the body's immune system, reduce inflammation, and promote healing. Here are some dietary recommendations to help fuel your body for healing plugged ducts:

1. Stay Hydrated: Staying hydrated is essential for breastfeeding mothers, as dehydration can lead to thicker, more concentrated milk that is more likely to clog ducts. Aim to drink at least 8-10 glasses of water per day, and consider adding in hydrating foods like fruits and vegetables.

2. Eat a Balanced Diet: A balanced diet rich in fruits, vegetables, whole grains, lean proteins, and healthy fats is essential for supporting your body's healing process. These foods provide essential nutrients like vitamins, minerals, and antioxidants that can help reduce inflammation and promote healing.

3. Include Foods Rich in Vitamin C: Vitamin C is a powerful antioxidant that can help boost the immune system and reduce inflammation. Include foods like oranges, strawberries, kiwi, bell peppers, and broccoli in your diet to help support healing.

4. Incorporate Omega-3 Fatty Acids: Omega-3 fatty acids are anti-inflammatory fats that can help reduce inflammation in the body. Include foods like salmon, walnuts, flaxseeds, and chia seeds in your diet to help support healing.

5. Avoid Foods that Can Increase Inflammation: Some foods can increase inflammation in the body, potentially worsening plugged ducts. Avoid foods high in sugar, refined carbohydrates, and trans fats, as these can contribute to inflammation. Instead, focus on whole, unprocessed foods to

support healing.

6. Consider Herbal Supplements: Some herbal supplements, like lecithin and sunflower lecithin, have been shown to help prevent and treat plugged ducts by reducing the stickiness of breast milk. Talk to a healthcare provider before starting any herbal supplements to ensure they are safe for you and your baby.

7. Don't Skip Meals: It's important to fuel your body with regular, balanced meals and snacks throughout the day. Skipping meals can lead to drops in blood sugar, which can impact milk production and increase the risk of plugged ducts. Aim to eat every 3-4 hours to keep your energy levels stable.

8. Practice Stress-Relief Techniques: Stress can impact milk production and increase the risk of plugged ducts. Incorporate stress-relief techniques like deep breathing, meditation, yoga, or gentle exercise into your daily

routine to help support healing.

9. Get Plenty of Rest: Rest is essential for healing, especially when dealing with plugged ducts. Aim to get 7-9 hours of sleep per night, and take breaks throughout the day to rest and recharge. Listen to your body and prioritize self-care during this time.

10. Seek Support: Dealing with plugged ducts can be challenging, both physically and emotionally. Reach out to a lactation consultant, healthcare provider, or support group for

guidance and encouragement. Having a strong support system can help you navigate this challenging time and support your healing journey.

In conclusion, nutrition plays a crucial role in healing plugged ducts.

By fueling your body with a balanced diet rich in essential nutrients, staying hydrated, and practicing self-care, you can support your body's healing process and reduce the risk of future plugged ducts.

Remember to listen to your body, seek support when needed, and prioritize self-care during this time. With the right nutrition and support, you can successfully navigate plugged ducts and continue to enjoy the breastfeeding journey with your baby.

The Role of Exercise in Preventing and Treating Plugged Ducts

Plugged ducts, also known as clogged ducts, are a common issue that can occur in breastfeeding mothers. They happen when milk ducts become blocked, preventing milk from flowing freely.

This can lead to pain, swelling, and even infection if not addressed promptly. While there are various factors that can contribute to plugged ducts, such as improper latch, infrequent feedings, or tight clothing, one often overlooked aspect is the role of exercise in preventing and treating plugged ducts.

Exercise is an essential component of overall health and well-being, and it can play a significant role in preventing and treating plugged ducts.

By incorporating regular physical activity into your routine, you can help improve circulation, reduce inflammation, and promote the flow of milk through your ducts.

In this article, we will explore the benefits of exercise for preventing and treating plugged ducts, as well as provide some tips on how to incorporate exercise into your daily life as a breastfeeding mother.

Preventing Plugged Ducts Through Exercise

Regular exercise can help prevent plugged ducts by improving circulation and reducing inflammation in the breast tissue. When you engage in physical activity, your heart rate increases, and blood flow to the breasts is enhanced. This increased circulation helps to keep the milk ducts clear and functioning properly, reducing the risk of blockages.

In addition to improving circulation, exercise can also help reduce inflammation in the breast tissue. Inflammation is a common factor in the development of plugged ducts, as it can cause the ducts to become swollen and constricted.

By engaging in regular physical activity, you can help to reduce inflammation in the breasts, making it less likely that a blockage will occur.

Furthermore, exercise can help to maintain a healthy weight, which is important for preventing plugged ducts. Excess weight can put added pressure on the milk ducts, making them more prone to blockages. By staying active and maintaining a healthy weight, you can reduce the risk of developing plugged ducts.

Tips for Preventing Plugged Ducts Through Exercise

To prevent plugged ducts through exercise, it is important to incorporate a variety of activities into your routine. Here are some tips to help you get started:

1. Choose activities that you enjoy: The key to sticking with an exercise routine is to choose activities that you enjoy. Whether

it's walking, swimming, yoga, or dancing, find something that you love to do and make it a regular part of your routine.

2. Stay active throughout the day: In addition to structured exercise, try to stay active throughout the day. Take breaks to stretch and move around, and incorporate physical activity into your daily tasks whenever possible.

3. Wear supportive clothing: When exercising, be sure to wear a supportive sports bra that provides proper support for your breasts. This can help to reduce strain on the milk ducts and prevent blockages.

4. Stay hydrated: It is important to stay hydrated while exercising, especially when breastfeeding. Drink plenty of water before, during, and after your workout to help keep your milk supply flowing smoothly.

Treating Plugged Ducts Through Exercise

If you do develop a plugged duct, exercise can also play a role in helping to treat the issue. By engaging in physical activity, you can help to loosen the blockage and promote the flow of milk through the affected duct. Exercise can also help to reduce pain and inflammation associated with plugged ducts, making it a valuable tool in the treatment process.

One effective exercise for treating plugged ducts is breast massage. Gently massaging the affected breast while exercising can help to break up the blockage and encourage the flow of milk. You can do this by using your fingers to apply gentle pressure in a circular motion around the blocked area.

In addition to breast massage, activities such as yoga and stretching can also be beneficial for treating plugged ducts. These exercises can help to improve flexibility and range of motion in the breast tissue, making it easier for milk to flow through the ducts. Gentle movements such as arm circles, shoulder rolls, and chest stretches can help to relieve pain and discomfort associated with plugged ducts.

Tips for Treating Plugged Ducts Through Exercise

If you are experiencing a plugged duct, here are some tips for using exercise to help treat the issue:

1. Start with gentle exercises: If you have a plugged duct, it is important to start with gentle exercises to avoid exacerbating the problem. Focus on activities that promote relaxation and gentle movement, such as yoga or walking.

2. Use heat therapy: Before exercising, apply a warm compress to the affected breast to help loosen the blockage. Heat therapy can help to reduce pain and inflammation, making it easier to exercise and massage the affected area.

Listen to your body: Pay attention to how your body is feeling while exercising. If you experience pain or discomfort, stop the activity   and   rest.

Chapter 6: Support Systems: Building a Strong Network for Plugged Duct Recovery

Breastfeeding can be a beautiful and rewarding experience for both mother and baby. However, it can also come with its challenges, one of which is dealing with plugged ducts.

A plugged duct occurs when a milk duct in the breast becomes blocked, causing milk to back up and create a painful lump.

This can be a frustrating and uncomfortable experience for breastfeeding mothers, but with the right support systems in place, it is possible to overcome plugged ducts and continue breastfeeding successfully.

One of the most important support systems for plugged duct recovery is having a strong network of people who can offer help and guidance.

This network can include healthcare providers, lactation consultants, support groups, and friends and family members who have experience with breastfeeding.

By building a strong network of support, breastfeeding mothers can access the resources and information they need to effectively manage plugged ducts and prevent them from reoccurring.

Healthcare providers play a crucial role in supporting breastfeeding mothers who are dealing with plugged ducts.

Obstetricians, pediatricians, and lactation consultants can provide valuable advice on how to relieve the pain and discomfort associated with plugged ducts, as well as offer tips on how to prevent them in the future.

Healthcare providers can also help mothers identify the underlying causes of plugged ducts, such as improper latch or infrequent nursing, and develop a plan to address these issues.

Lactation consultants are particularly valuable resources for breastfeeding mothers struggling with plugged ducts. These professionals are trained to provide expert guidance on breastfeeding techniques, proper positioning, and other strategies for managing common breastfeeding challenges. Lactation consultants can also offer emotional support and reassurance to mothers who may be feeling overwhelmed or discouraged by their plugged ducts.

Support groups are another important component of a strong support network for plugged duct recovery. These groups provide a safe and nonjudgmental space for breastfeeding mothers to share their experiences, ask questions, and seek advice from others who have been through similar challenges.

Support groups can be in- person or online, and they can be a valuable source of information and encouragement for mothers dealing with plugged ducts.

Friends and family members can also play a key role in supporting breastfeeding mothers during plugged duct recovery.

Loved ones can offer practical help, such as preparing meals or caring for older children, to give mothers the time and space they need to focus on their breastfeeding journey.

Friends and family members can also provide emotional support and encouragement, helping mothers stay positive and motivated as they work through the challenges of plugged ducts.

In addition to building a strong support network, there are several practical strategies that breastfeeding mothers can use to manage plugged ducts and promote recovery.

One of the most effective ways to relieve a plugged duct is through frequent nursing or pumping. By emptying the affected breast regularly, mothers can help to clear the blockage and reduce pain and swelling.

Warm compresses, gentle massage, and hot showers can also be helpful in alleviating discomfort and promoting milk flow.

It is also important for breastfeeding mothers to prioritize self-care during plugged duct recovery. This may include getting plenty of rest, staying hydrated, and eating a balanced diet rich in nutrients that support breastfeeding. Mothers should also pay attention to their own comfort and well-being, taking breaks when needed and seeking help from their support network when they are feeling overwhelmed.

In some cases, plugged ducts may require medical intervention to resolve. If a plugged duct does not improve with home remedies and self-care, healthcare providers may recommend treatments such as prescription medications or ultrasound therapy to help clear the blockage.

It is important for mothers to communicate openly with their healthcare providers about their symptoms and concerns, so that they can receive the appropriate care and support for plugged duct recovery.

Overall, building a strong support network is essential for breastfeeding mothers who are dealing with plugged ducts.

By connecting with healthcare providers, lactation consultants, support groups, and loved ones, mothers can access the resources and encouragement they need to effectively manage plugged ducts and continue breastfeeding successfully.

With the right support systems in place, breastfeeding mothers can overcome the challenges of plugged ducts and enjoy a positive and fulfilling breastfeeding experience with their baby.

Rest and Recovery: The Importance of Self-Care for Plugged Ducts Rest

Breastfeeding is a beautiful and natural process that provides numerous benefits for both mother and baby. However, it can also come with its own set of challenges, one of which is plugged ducts.

Plugged ducts occur when milk flow is obstructed in a milk duct, causing pain, swelling, and inflammation in the affected breast.

This can be a painful and frustrating experience for breastfeeding mothers, but with the right self-care practices, plugged ducts can be effectively managed and resolved.

One of the most important aspects of self-care for plugged ducts is rest and recovery. Resting and taking care of yourself is crucial for your overall health and well-being, especially when dealing with a plugged duct.

In this article, we will explore the importance of rest and recovery for plugged ducts and provide tips on how to incorporate self-care practices into your daily routine.

Importance of Rest and Recovery for Plugged Ducts

Rest and recovery play a crucial role in the management and resolution of plugged ducts. When you are experiencing a plugged duct, your body is already under stress and inflammation, and not giving yourself the time and space to rest and recover can exacerbate the situation. Here are some reasons why rest and recovery are essential for plugged ducts:

1. Promotes Healing: Resting allows your body to focus on healing the affected breast and resolving the plugged duct. When you are constantly on the go and not giving your body the time it needs to recover, it can prolong the healing process and make the plugged duct more difficult to resolve.

2. Reduces Inflammation: Plugged ducts are often accompanied by inflammation in the affected breast, which can cause pain and discomfort. Resting and taking care of yourself can help reduce inflammation and alleviate symptoms associated with plugged ducts.

3. Prevents Complications: Ignoring the signs of a plugged duct and not taking the time to rest and recover can lead to complications such as mastitis, a more serious condition that requires medical intervention.

By prioritizing rest and recovery, you can prevent the development of complications and promote a faster resolution of the plugged duct.

4. Supports Milk Supply: Resting and taking care of yourself can also help support your milk supply. Stress and fatigue can negatively impact milk production, so it is important to prioritize self-care practices to ensure that you are able to

continue breastfeeding successfully.

Tips for Incorporating Self-Care Practices into Your Routine

Now that we have established the importance of rest and recovery for plugged ducts, let's explore some tips on how to incorporate self-care practices into your daily routine:

1. Prioritize Sleep: Getting an adequate amount of sleep is essential for rest and recovery, especially when dealing with a plugged duct. Aim to get at least 7-8 hours of sleep each night to support your body's healing process.

2. Stay Hydrated: Drinking plenty of water is important for overall health and can help prevent dehydration, which can contribute to the development of plugged ducts. Aim to drink at least 8-10 glasses of water each day to stay hydrated.

3. Practice Gentle Breast Massage: Massaging the affected breast can help promote milk flow and alleviate symptoms of a plugged duct. Use gentle circular motions to massage the breast before and after breastfeeding to help clear the obstruction.

4. Apply Heat: Applying heat to the affected breast can help reduce inflammation and promote milk flow. Use a warm compress or take a warm shower before breastfeeding to help loosen the plugged duct.

5. Take Breaks: It is important to listen to your body and take

breaks when needed. If you are feeling fatigued or in pain, take a break from your daily activities and focus on resting and recovering.

6. Seek Support: Reach out to a lactation consultant or healthcare provider for support and guidance on managing plugged ducts. They can provide additional resources and recommendations to help you effectively resolve the issue.

7. Practice Self-Care: Take time for yourself and engage in activities that bring you joy and relaxation. Whether it's reading a book, taking a walk, or practicing mindfulness, prioritize self-care practices to support your overall well-being.

In conclusion, rest and recovery are essential components of self-care for plugged ducts. By prioritizing rest, staying hydrated, practicing gentle breast massage, applying heat, taking breaks, seeking support, and practicing self-care, you can effectively manage and resolve plugged ducts.

Remember to listen to your body and give yourself the time and space you need to heal and recover. Breastfeeding is a journey that requires patience and self-care, and by incorporating these practices into your routine, you can navigate the challenges of plugged ducts with confidence and ease.

Embracing Change: Adapting Your Routine for Plugged Duct Relief Embracing Change

Breastfeeding is a beautiful and natural process that provides numerous benefits for both mother and baby. However, it is not without its challenges. One common issue that many breastfeeding mothers face is plugged ducts.

A plugged duct occurs when a milk duct becomes blocked, leading to a painful lump in the breast. This can be a frustrating and uncomfortable experience, but there are steps you can take to relieve the pain and prevent future occurrences.

One of the most important things you can do to prevent plugged ducts is to ensure that you have a good breastfeeding routine. This includes feeding your baby frequently and on demand, as well as making sure that you are emptying your breasts completely during each feeding.

However, even with a good routine in place, plugged ducts can still occur. When they do, it is important to take action quickly to relieve the pain and prevent further complications.

One of the most effective ways to relieve a plugged duct is to apply heat to the affected area. This can help to loosen the blockage and encourage the milk to flow more freely. You can do this by taking a warm shower or bath, using a warm compress, or even applying a heating pad to the affected breast. Massaging the area gently while applying heat can also help to break up the blockage and relieve the pain.

Another important step in relieving a plugged duct is to ensure that you are nursing your baby frequently and on demand. This can help to keep the milk flowing and prevent further blockages from occurring.

If your baby is having trouble latching or nursing effectively, you may need to seek help from a lactation consultant or other breastfeeding support professional. They can help you to address any issues that may be contributing to the plugged duct and provide guidance on how to improve your breastfeeding technique.

In addition to nursing frequently, it is also important to ensure that you are using proper breastfeeding positions. This can help to ensure that your baby is able to latch properly and empty your breasts completely during each feeding.

Experimenting with different positions, such as the football hold or side-lying position, can help to relieve pressure on the affected duct and encourage the milk to flow more freely.

It is also important to stay hydrated and well-nourished while breastfeeding. Drinking plenty of water and eating a balanced diet can help to keep your milk supply flowing and prevent blockages from occurring. If you are experiencing frequent plugged ducts, you may want to consider adding foods that are known to support milk production, such as oatmeal, flaxseeds, and leafy greens, to your diet.

In some cases, over-the-counter pain relievers may be necessary to help manage the discomfort associated with a plugged duct.

However, it is important to consult with your healthcare provider before taking any medication while breastfeeding, as some medications can pass through breast milk to your baby.

Your healthcare provider can help you to determine the safest and most effective treatment options for your specific situation.

If you are unable to relieve the pain and discomfort of a plugged duct on your own, it may be necessary to seek medical intervention.

Your healthcare provider may recommend using a breast pump to help empty the affected breast more effectively, or they may recommend a procedure called ultrasound-guided aspiration to remove the blockage. In severe cases, surgery may be necessary to address a persistent or recurrent plugged duct.

While dealing with a plugged duct can be a challenging and frustrating experience, it is important to remember that it is a common issue that many breastfeeding mothers face. By taking proactive steps to prevent blockages from occurring and seeking help when needed, you can effectively manage plugged ducts and continue to enjoy the many benefits of breastfeeding.

In conclusion, embracing change and adapting your routine for plugged duct relief is essential for maintaining a healthy breastfeeding relationship with your baby.

By following the tips and strategies outlined in this article, you can effectively manage plugged ducts and prevent future occurrences.

Remember to stay hydrated, nurse frequently, use proper breastfeeding positions, and seek help when needed. With the right support and guidance, you can overcome the challenges of plugged ducts and continue to enjoy the many benefits of breastfeeding for both you and your baby.

Chapter 7: Overcoming Challenges: Strategies for Dealing with Stubborn Plugged Ducts

Breastfeeding is a wonderful and natural way to nourish your baby, but it can come with its fair share of challenges. One common issue that many breastfeeding mothers face is dealing with stubborn plugged ducts.

A plugged duct occurs when a milk duct in the breast becomes blocked, leading to a build-up of milk that can cause pain, swelling, and inflammation. If left untreated, a plugged duct can lead to a more serious condition known as mastitis, which is an infection of the breast tissue.

Dealing with stubborn plugged ducts can be frustrating and painful, but there are strategies that you can use to overcome this common breastfeeding challenge. In this article, we will discuss some effective ways to deal with stubborn plugged ducts and prevent them from recurring in the future.

1. Identify the Symptoms

The first step in dealing with a plugged duct is to identify the symptoms. Some common signs of a plugged duct include:

- Pain or tenderness in one breast
- A hard lump or swelling in the breast
- Redness or warmth in the affected area
- Decreased milk supply from the affected breast
- Fever or flu-like symptoms

If you are experiencing any of these symptoms, it is important to take action right away to prevent the plugged duct from turning into mastitis. The sooner you address the issue, the easier it will be to resolve.

2. Nurse Frequently and on Demand

One of the most effective ways to clear a plugged duct is to nurse frequently and on demand. The more often you empty your breast, the less likely it is that a blockage will occur.

Make sure to nurse your baby on both breasts during each feeding session, even if one breast is affected by a plugged duct. This will help to prevent further build-up of milk in the affected breast.

If your baby is having trouble latching onto the affected breast due to the pain or swelling, try different breastfeeding positions to find one that is more comfortable for both of you. You can also try using a breast pump to help empty the affected breast if nursing alone is not effective.

3. Apply Heat and Massage

Another effective strategy for dealing with stubborn plugged ducts is to apply heat and massage to the affected breast. Heat can help to loosen up the blockage and improve milk flow, while massage can help to break up the blockage and promote drainage.

You can apply heat to the affected breast by taking a warm shower or bath, using a heating pad or warm compress, or placing a warm washcloth on the breast.

Massage the affected breast gently in a circular motion towards the nipple to help move the blockage towards the milk duct opening. You can also try hand expressing some milk from the affected breast to help relieve the pressure and pain.

4. Stay Hydrated and Rest

It is important to stay hydrated and get plenty of rest when dealing with a plugged duct. Drinking plenty of water will help to thin out your breast milk and make it easier to flow, while getting enough rest will help your body to heal and recover more quickly.

Make sure to drink at least 8-10 glasses of water a day to stay hydrated and support your milk supply. You can also try drinking herbal teas such as fenugreek or blessed thistle to help increase your milk production. Getting plenty of rest and taking breaks throughout the day to relax and unwind will also help to reduce stress and promote healing.

5. Use Natural Remedies

There are several natural remedies that you can use to help clear a stubborn plugged duct. Some effective remedies include:

- Epsom salt soak: Soaking your affected breast in warm water mixed with Epsom salt can help to reduce inflammation and promote drainage.

- Cabbage leaves: Applying cold cabbage leaves to the affected breast can help to reduce swelling and pain.
- Essential oils: Massaging the affected breast with essential oils such as lavender or tea tree oil can help to reduce inflammation and promote healing.

Before using any natural remedies, make sure to consult with your healthcare provider to ensure that they are safe for you and your baby. It is also important to use these remedies in conjunction with other strategies for dealing with plugged ducts, such as nursing frequently and applying heat and massage.

6. Seek Professional Help

If you have tried all of the above strategies and are still experiencing stubborn plugged ducts, it may be time to seek professional help. Your healthcare provider or lactation consultant can help to assess the situation and provide you with personalized advice and treatment options.

In some cases, your healthcare provider may recommend using a prescription medication such as an antibiotic or anti-inflammatory to help clear the plugged duct. They may also recommend using a hospital-grade breast pump to help empty the affected breast more effectively.

If you are experiencing severe pain, fever, or other symptoms of mastitis, it is important to seek medical attention right away. Mastitis is a serious condition that requires prompt treatment with antibiotics to prevent further complications.

The Emotional Impact of Plugged Ducts: Navigating Feelings of Frustration and Guilt

Breastfeeding is a beautiful and natural process that provides numerous benefits to both the mother and the baby. However, it is not always smooth sailing, and many mothers may encounter challenges along the way.

One common issue that breastfeeding mothers may face is plugged ducts, which can be painful and frustrating to deal with.

In addition to the physical discomfort, plugged ducts can also have a significant emotional impact on mothers, leading to feelings of frustration and guilt.

Plugged ducts occur when a milk duct in the breast becomes blocked, preventing milk from flowing freely. This blockage can be caused by a variety of factors, including improper latching, infrequent feedings, tight clothing, or even stress.

When a duct becomes plugged, it can lead to pain, swelling, and inflammation in the affected breast. In severe cases, a plugged duct can progress to mastitis, a more serious condition that requires medical treatment.

Dealing with plugged ducts can be a frustrating experience for many mothers. The pain and discomfort that come with a plugged duct can make breastfeeding a painful and unpleasant experience. Mothers may also feel frustrated that their bodies are not functioning as they should, leading to feelings of inadequacy and self-doubt.

Additionally, the physical discomfort of a plugged duct can make it difficult for mothers to care for their babies and perform daily tasks, adding to their feelings of frustration and helplessness.

In addition to frustration, mothers may also experience feelings of guilt when dealing with plugged ducts. Many mothers feel guilty that they are not able to provide their babies with the nourishment they need, or that they are not living up to the ideal of the perfect mother.

This guilt can be exacerbated by societal pressure to breastfeed exclusively and the belief that breastfeeding is the best and only way to feed a baby.

Mothers may also feel guilty for experiencing negative emotions about breastfeeding, as they may feel that they should be grateful for the opportunity to breastfeed their babies.

Navigating these feelings of frustration and guilt can be challenging for mothers dealing with plugged ducts. It is important for mothers to remember that plugged ducts are a common and normal occurrence in breastfeeding, and that they are not a reflection of their abilities as a mother. Seeking support from healthcare providers, lactation consultants, and other mothers who have experienced plugged ducts can help mothers feel less alone and more empowered to overcome this challenge.

In addition to seeking support, there are several strategies that mothers can use to help prevent and manage plugged ducts.

Ensuring proper latching and positioning during breastfeeding, feeding frequently, wearing loose- fitting clothing, and applying heat and massage to the affected breast can all help to prevent and alleviate plugged ducts.

If a plugged duct does occur, continuing to breastfeed on the affected side, massaging the breast, and applying heat can help to clear the blockage and relieve discomfort.

It is also important for mothers to take care of themselves emotionally while dealing with plugged ducts. Practicing self-care, such as getting enough rest, eating well, and engaging in activities that bring joy and relaxation, can help mothers cope with the emotional toll of dealing with plugged ducts.

 It is also important for mothers to be gentle with themselves and to remember that it is okay to feel frustrated and guilty at times.
Seeking professional help from a therapist or counselor can also be beneficial for mothers who are struggling to cope with their emotions.

In conclusion, plugged ducts can have a significant emotional impact on breastfeeding mothers, leading to feelings of frustration and guilt. It is important for mothers to seek support, practice self-care, and use strategies to prevent and manage plugged ducts.

By taking care of themselves emotionally and physically, mothers can navigate the challenges of plugged ducts and continue to provide their babies with the nourishment and love they need. Remember, you are not alone in this journey, and there is help and support available to help you through this challenging time.

Empowering Yourself: Taking Control of Your Plugged Duct

Breastfeeding is a beautiful and natural process that provides numerous benefits to both the mother and the baby. However, it is not without its challenges.

One common issue that many breastfeeding mothers face is plugged ducts. A plugged duct occurs when a milk duct in the breast becomes blocked, leading to discomfort, pain, and potential complications if not addressed promptly.

Plugged ducts can be caused by a variety of factors, including inadequate milk removal, improper latching, tight clothing, or even stress.

Regardless of the cause, dealing with a plugged duct can be frustrating and overwhelming for many mothers. However, it is important to remember that you are not alone in this journey, and there are steps you can take to empower yourself and take control of your plugged duct journey.

In this article, we will discuss some practical tips and strategies to help you navigate through the challenges of dealing with plugged ducts. By empowering yourself with knowledge and resources, you can effectively address plugged ducts and continue to enjoy the benefits of breastfeeding your baby.

Understanding Plugged Ducts

Before we delve into how to empower yourself in dealing with plugged ducts, let's first understand what a plugged duct is and how it can impact your breastfeeding journey.

A plugged duct occurs when a milk duct in the breast becomes blocked, preventing the flow of milk. This blockage can lead to a build-up of milk, inflammation, and pain in the affected area.

Common symptoms of a plugged duct include:

- A tender or painful lump in the breast
- Redness or swelling in the affected area
- A feeling of fullness or heaviness in the breast
- Discomfort or pain while breastfeeding
- Flu-like symptoms, such as fever or chills

It is important to address a plugged duct promptly to prevent further complications, such as mastitis, a more serious condition that can result from untreated plugged ducts.

Mastitis is characterized by inflammation and infection of the breast tissue, leading to more severe symptoms and potentially requiring medical intervention.

Empowering Yourself: Practical Tips and Strategies

Dealing with a plugged duct can be challenging, but there are steps you can take to empower yourself and take control of your plugged duct journey. By arming yourself with knowledge and resources, you can effectively address plugged ducts and continue to breastfeed your baby with confidence. Here are some practical tips and strategies to help you navigate through the challenges of dealing with plugged ducts:

1. Educate Yourself

One of the most important steps in empowering yourself in dealing with plugged ducts is to educate yourself

about the condition. Learn about the causes of plugged ducts, common symptoms, and effective treatment options. Understanding how plugged ducts occur and how they can impact your breastfeeding journey will help you feel more confident in addressing the issue when it arises.

There are numerous resources available online, such as reputable websites, breastfeeding support groups, and lactation consultants, that can provide valuable information and guidance on dealing with plugged ducts. Take the time to research and educate yourself about plugged ducts to empower yourself in managing the condition effectively.

2. Maintain Good Breastfeeding Practices

Prevention is key when it comes to dealing with plugged ducts. By maintaining good breastfeeding practices, you can reduce the risk of developing plugged ducts and ensure optimal milk flow. Some tips for preventing plugged ducts include:

- Ensure proper latching and positioning while breastfeeding

- Feed your baby frequently to prevent engorgement
- Use a breast pump or hand expression to fully empty your breasts
- Avoid tight clothing or bras that can constrict milk flow
- Practice good hygiene by keeping your breasts clean and dry

By incorporating these practices into your breastfeeding routine, you can minimize the likelihood of developing plugged ducts and promote healthy milk flow in your breasts.

3. Address Plugged Ducts Promptly

If you do experience a plugged duct, it is important to address it promptly to prevent further complications. Some effective strategies for resolving plugged ducts include:

- Apply warm compresses to the affected area to help reduce inflammation and promote milk flow

- Massage the affected breast gently to help release the blockage
- Nurse or pump frequently to empty the breast and relieve pressure

- Take over-the-counter pain relievers, such as ibuprofen, to alleviate discomfort

- Rest and stay hydrated to support your body's healing process
  If you are unable to resolve a plugged duct on your own or if you develop symptoms of mastitis, such as a high fever or worsening pain, seek medical attention immediately.

Your healthcare provider can provide additional support and treatment options to help you recover from a plugged duct and prevent further complications.

4. Seek Support

Dealing with plugged ducts can be emotionally and physically taxing, especially for new mothers.

Chapter 8: The Healing Power of Nature: Harnessing Earth's Remedies for Plugged Duct Relief

Breastfeeding is a beautiful and natural way to nourish your baby, but it can also come with its challenges. One common issue that many breastfeeding mothers face is plugged ducts.

These painful blockages can occur when milk is not properly draining from the breast, leading to a buildup of milk that can cause inflammation and discomfort.

While there are conventional treatments for plugged ducts, such as warm compresses, massage, and frequent nursing, some mothers may be interested in exploring more natural remedies.

The healing power of nature offers a variety of remedies that can help to relieve plugged ducts and promote healing in the breast tissue.

One of the most well-known natural remedies for plugged ducts is the use of cabbage leaves. Cabbage leaves have been used for centuries as a remedy for breast engorgement and plugged ducts.

Simply take a few cabbage leaves, wash them thoroughly, and place them in your bra over the affected breast. The coolness of the cabbage leaves can help to reduce inflammation and promote drainage of the milk ducts.

Another natural remedy for plugged ducts is the use of essential oils. Lavender, peppermint, and eucalyptus essential oils are known for their anti-inflammatory and pain-relieving properties.

You can dilute a few drops of these oils in a carrier oil, such as coconut or almond oil, and massage them into the affected breast. This can help to reduce inflammation and promote healing in the breast tissue.

Herbal remedies can also be effective in relieving plugged ducts. Fenugreek, blessed thistle, and red clover are all herbs that are known for their ability to increase milk production and promote healthy breastfeeding.

You can find these herbs in supplement form or as teas, and incorporate them into your daily routine to help prevent plugged ducts from occurring.

In addition to these natural remedies, there are also lifestyle changes that can help to prevent plugged ducts. Ensuring proper hydration, maintaining a healthy diet, and getting plenty of rest can all help to promote healthy breastfeeding and prevent blockages in the milk ducts.

It is also important to ensure that your baby is latching properly and nursing frequently to help prevent plugged ducts from occurring.

While natural remedies can be effective in relieving plugged ducts, it is important to consult with a healthcare provider before trying any new treatment. Plugged ducts can lead to more serious issues, such as mastitis, if not properly treated.

Your healthcare provider can help to determine the best course of treatment for your individual situation and ensure that you and your baby remain healthy and happy.

In conclusion, the healing power of nature offers a variety of remedies that can help to relieve plugged ducts and promote healing in the breast tissue.

From cabbage leaves to essential oils to herbal supplements, there are many natural remedies that can help to prevent and treat plugged ducts.

By incorporating these remedies into your daily routine and making healthy lifestyle choices, you can help to ensure a smooth and comfortable breastfeeding experience for you and your baby.

Mind-Body Connection: How Mental Health Affects Plugged Ducts

The mind-body connection is a powerful and often overlooked aspect of our overall health and well-being. Our mental health can have a significant impact on various physical aspects of our bodies, including the development of plugged ducts.

Plugged ducts are a common issue for many breastfeeding mothers, and they can be painful and frustrating to deal with. Understanding the connection between mental health and plugged ducts can help us better manage and prevent this issue.

Plugged ducts occur when milk ducts in the breast become blocked, preventing milk from flowing freely. This can lead to a build-up of milk, inflammation, and pain in the affected area.

Plugged ducts can be caused by a variety of factors, including improper breastfeeding techniques, tight clothing, and stress. The relationship between mental health and plugged ducts lies in the impact that stress and anxiety can have on the body.

Stress and anxiety can cause the body to produce higher levels of cortisol, a hormone that can affect the immune system and inflammation response. When stress levels are high, the body may be more prone to inflammation and blockages in the milk ducts. Additionally, stress can also affect breastfeeding patterns and techniques, leading to a higher risk of plugged ducts.

Furthermore, stress and anxiety can also impact the let-down reflex, which is the process by which milk is released from the breast during breastfeeding.

When a mother is stressed or anxious, her body may not release milk as effectively, leading to a higher likelihood of plugged ducts. It is essential for breastfeeding mothers to prioritize their mental health and well-being to reduce the risk of developing plugged ducts.

In addition to stress and anxiety, other mental health issues can also contribute to plugged ducts. Postpartum depression, for example, can affect a mother's ability to breastfeed effectively and may lead to irregular feeding patterns that increase the risk of plugged ducts.

It is crucial for mothers experiencing postpartum depression to seek support and treatment to manage their mental health and reduce the risk of plugged ducts.

It is essential for breastfeeding mothers to prioritize self-care and mental health to reduce the risk of developing plugged ducts.

Practicing relaxation techniques, such as deep breathing exercises or meditation, can help reduce stress levels and promote a healthy breastfeeding experience. Additionally, seeking support from healthcare providers, lactation consultants, or support groups can provide valuable resources and guidance for managing mental health and breastfeeding challenges.

Incorporating self-care practices into daily routines can also help prevent plugged ducts and promote overall well- being. Eating a balanced diet, staying hydrated, and getting regular exercise can support milk production and reduce the risk of inflammation in the milk ducts.

Taking breaks, getting enough rest, and seeking help with household tasks can also help reduce stress levels and support mental health during the breastfeeding journey.

Furthermore, communication and support from partners, family members, and friends can play a crucial role in promoting mental health and preventing plugged ducts.

Partners can offer emotional support, assist with breastfeeding tasks, and provide encouragement during challenging times.

Family members and friends can help with childcare, household chores, and meal preparation to reduce the burden on breastfeeding mothers and promote a positive mental state.

In conclusion, the mind-body connection plays a significant role in the development of plugged ducts in breastfeeding mothers. Stress, anxiety, and other mental health issues can impact milk production, breastfeeding techniques, and inflammation in the milk ducts, leading to a higher risk of plugged ducts. Prioritizing mental health, self-care, and support can help reduce the risk of plugged ducts and promote a positive breastfeeding experience.

By understanding the connection between mental health and plugged ducts, breastfeeding mothers can take proactive steps to support their well-being and prevent this common issue.

Finding Joy in the Journey: Celebrating Small Victories with Plugged Duct Relief

Finding joy in the journey of motherhood can be a challenging task, especially when faced with common issues such as plugged ducts while breastfeeding.

However, celebrating small victories along the way can make the experience more fulfilling and rewarding. In this article, we will explore the importance of finding joy in the journey of motherhood, how to overcome plugged ducts, and the significance of celebrating small victories in the process.

Motherhood is a journey filled with ups and downs, challenges and triumphs. From the moment a woman discovers she is pregnant, to the day she holds her newborn in her arms, the journey is a rollercoaster of emotions and experiences.

While the joy of bringing new life into the world is unparalleled, there are also moments of doubt, frustration, and exhaustion. One common challenge that many breastfeeding mothers face is plugged ducts.

Plugged ducts occur when milk is not effectively removed from the breast, leading to a blockage in the milk duct. This can cause pain, swelling, and inflammation in the affected breast, making breastfeeding uncomfortable and challenging. Plugged ducts can be caused by a variety of factors, including improper latching, infrequent feedings, tight clothing, and stress.

While plugged ducts are a common issue among breastfeeding mothers, they can be overcome with the right strategies and support.

One of the key ways to overcome plugged ducts is to ensure proper breastfeeding techniques. This includes ensuring a proper latch, feeding on demand, and using different breastfeeding positions to effectively drain the breast.

Massage and warm compresses can also help to relieve the blockage and promote milk flow. In some cases, a breastfeeding counselor or lactation consultant may be able to provide additional support and guidance.

In addition to addressing the physical symptoms of plugged ducts, it is also important for breastfeeding mothers to take care of their emotional well-being.

The stress and discomfort of dealing with plugged ducts can take a toll on a mother's mental health, leading to feelings of frustration, guilt, and inadequacy. It is important for mothers to seek support from their partners, family members, and healthcare providers to help them navigate this challenging time.

Finding joy in the journey of motherhood involves celebrating small victories along the way. While overcoming plugged ducts may seem like a small feat in the grand scheme of motherhood, it is important to acknowledge and celebrate each success, no matter how small.

Whether it's successfully clearing a plugged duct, increasing milk supply, or mastering a new breastfeeding position, every victory is a step towards a healthier and happier breastfeeding journey.

One way to celebrate small victories in the journey of motherhood is to keep a journal or diary of your breastfeeding experiences.

Write down your thoughts, feelings, and accomplishments, no matter how insignificant they may seem. Reflecting on your journey and acknowledging your progress can help to boost your confidence and motivation to continue breastfeeding, even in the face of challenges.

Another way to celebrate small victories is to share your successes with others. Joining a breastfeeding support group or online community can provide you with a network of like-minded mothers who can offer advice, encouragement, and support.

Sharing your experiences and triumphs with others can help to normalize the challenges of breastfeeding and remind you that you are not alone in your journey.

In addition to finding joy in the journey of motherhood, it is also important to take care of yourself during this time. Remember to prioritize self-care, get plenty of rest, eat a healthy diet, and stay hydrated.

 Taking care of yourself will not only benefit your physical and mental health but also help to ensure a successful breastfeeding journey.

In conclusion, finding joy in the journey of motherhood is a rewarding and fulfilling experience, despite the challenges and obstacles that may arise along the way.

By overcoming plugged ducts, celebrating small victories, and taking care of yourself, you can navigate the ups and downs of breastfeeding with confidence and resilience. Remember that every breastfeeding journey is unique, and it's okay to ask for help and support when needed.

Celebrate your successes, no matter how small, and cherish the precious moments of motherhood.

Chapter 9: Beyond the Pain: Rediscovering Comfort and Ease with Plugged Ducts Beyond the Pain

Breastfeeding is a beautiful and natural way to nourish your baby, but it can also come with its fair share of challenges. One common issue that many breastfeeding mothers face is plugged ducts.

Plugged ducts occur when milk ducts in the breast become blocked, leading to pain, discomfort, and potential complications if not addressed promptly.

In this article, we will explore the causes of plugged ducts, how to prevent them, and effective ways to treat them so that you can continue breastfeeding with comfort and ease.

What Causes Plugged Ducts?

Plugged ducts can occur for a variety of reasons, but some common causes include:

- Infrequent or irregular breastfeeding or pumping: When milk is not regularly and effectively removed from the breast, it can accumulate and lead to a blockage in the milk ducts.

- Pressure on the breast: Wearing tight clothing, using a poorly fitting bra, or sleeping in a position that puts pressure on the breast can also contribute to plugged ducts.

- Stress or fatigue: Emotional stress, lack of sleep, or other factors that compromise your immune system can make you more susceptible to developing plugged ducts.

- Poor latch or positioning: If your baby is not latching properly or if you are not positioning them correctly during breastfeeding, it can lead to incomplete milk removal and the development of plugged ducts.

- Mastitis: Plugged ducts can sometimes be a precursor to mastitis, a more serious condition that involves inflammation and infection of the breast tissue.

How to Prevent Plugged Ducts

While plugged ducts can be uncomfortable and disruptive, there are steps you can take to help prevent them from occurring in the first place. Here are some tips for maintaining healthy breasts and milk ducts:

- Breastfeed frequently: The more often you breastfeed your baby, the less likely you are to develop plugged ducts. Aim to breastfeed at least every 2-3 hours during the day and once or twice at night.

- Ensure a proper latch: Make sure your baby is latching

correctly and effectively emptying the breast during feedings. If you are experiencing pain or discomfort while breastfeeding, seek help from a lactation consultant or healthcare provider.

- Avoid tight clothing: Wear loose-fitting, comfortable clothing that does not put pressure on your breasts. Avoid underwire bras and tight sports bras that can constrict milk flow.

- Stay hydrated: Drink plenty of water throughout the day to help maintain good milk production and prevent dehydration, which can contribute to plugged ducts.

- Rest and relax: Take time to rest and relax, especially in the early postpartum period when your body is adjusting to the demands of breastfeeding. Practice self-care activities that help reduce stress and promote relaxation.

- Use heat and massage: Applying warm compresses to your breasts before feeding can help loosen any blockages in the milk ducts. Gentle massage while breastfeeding can also help improve milk flow and prevent plugged ducts.

- Change breastfeeding positions: Experiment with different breastfeeding positions to ensure that your baby is effectively draining all areas of the breast. Side-lying, football hold, and laid-back breastfeeding positions can be helpful for preventing plugged ducts.

How to Treat Plugged Ducts

If you do develop a plugged duct, it is important to address it promptly to prevent it from progressing to mastitis or other complications. Here are some effective ways to treat plugged ducts and find relief from pain and discomfort:

- Nurse frequently: Breastfeed your baby as often as possible, starting with the affected breast. The suction and pressure from nursing can help to dislodge the blockage and promote milk flow.

- Apply heat: Use warm compresses or take a warm shower before breastfeeding to help soften the blockage and improve milk flow. You can also use a heating pad or warm rice sock on the affected breast between feedings.

- Massage the affected area: Gently massage the area of the breast where the blockage is located, using circular motions and light pressure. This can help to break up the blockage and encourage milk to flow more freely.

- Ensure proper drainage: Make sure your baby is latching correctly and effectively emptying the breast during feedings. If necessary, pump after breastfeeding to fully empty the breast and prevent further blockages.

- Rest and hydrate: Take time to rest and care for yourself while you are treating a plugged duct. Stay hydrated and nourished to support your body's healing process.

- Use over-the-counter remedies: Some breastfeeding mothers find relief from plugged ducts by taking over-the- counter pain relievers such as ibuprofen or acetaminophen. These medications can help reduce inflammation and alleviate discomfort.

- Consult a healthcare provider: If you are unable to resolve the plugged duct on your own or if you develop symptoms of mastitis, such as fever, chills, or redness of the

The Art of Self-Compassion: Practicing Kindness in the Face of Plugged Duct Challenges

Self-compassion is a powerful tool that can help individuals navigate through challenging situations with kindness and understanding.

When faced with plugged duct challenges while breastfeeding, practicing self- compassion can make a significant difference in how one copes with the situation.

Breastfeeding is a natural and beautiful experience that allows mothers to bond with their babies while providing them with essential nutrients. However, it can also come with its own set of challenges, one of which is plugged ducts.

A plugged duct occurs when a milk duct becomes blocked, causing milk to back up and create a painful lump in the breast.

This can be a frustrating and uncomfortable experience for mothers, but practicing self- compassion can help make the situation more manageable.

Self-compassion involves treating oneself with the same kindness and understanding that one would offer to a friend in a similar situation. It involves acknowledging one's pain and suffering without judgment, and offering oneself words of comfort and encouragement. When faced with plugged duct challenges, practicing self- compassion can help mothers cope with the physical discomfort and emotional stress that comes with the situation.

One way to practice self-compassion in the face of plugged duct challenges is to acknowledge and validate one's feelings. It is normal to feel frustrated, overwhelmed, and even guilty when dealing with breastfeeding difficulties.

Instead of suppressing these emotions, it is important to acknowledge them and recognize that they are a natural response to a challenging situation.

By allowing oneself to feel and express these emotions, one can begin to process them and move towards a place of healing and acceptance.

Another way to practice self-compassion in the face of plugged duct challenges is to practice self-care. This can involve taking time to rest, relax, and engage in activities that bring joy and comfort.

It can also involve seeking support from loved ones, healthcare providers, or lactation consultants who can offer guidance and assistance.

By prioritizing one's own well-being and seeking help when needed, mothers can better cope with the physical and emotional demands of dealing with plugged ducts.

In addition to acknowledging and validating one's feelings, and practicing self-care, self-compassion also involves practicing self-kindness.

This means treating oneself with gentleness and understanding, even when faced with challenges or setbacks. Instead of berating oneself for not being able to breastfeed as smoothly as one had hoped, it is important to offer oneself words of encouragement and support.

By speaking to oneself in a compassionate and loving manner, mothers can build resilience and strength in the face of plugged duct challenges.

Practicing self-compassion in the face of plugged duct challenges can also involve cultivating a sense of mindfulness.

Mindfulness involves being present in the moment and observing one's thoughts and feelings without judgment. By practicing mindfulness, mothers can become more aware of their reactions to plugged duct challenges and learn to respond to them with kindness and compassion.

This can help reduce stress and anxiety, and promote a sense of calm and balance in the midst of difficult circumstances.

In addition to practicing self-compassion, mothers dealing with plugged duct challenges can also benefit from seeking professional help and support. Lactation consultants, healthcare providers, and breastfeeding support groups can offer guidance, advice, and encouragement to help mothers navigate through the challenges of breastfeeding.

By reaching out for help and support, mothers can gain valuable insights and resources to help them overcome plugged duct challenges and continue breastfeeding successfully.

Overall, the art of self-compassion is a powerful tool that can help mothers navigate through plugged duct challenges with kindness and understanding.

By acknowledging and validating one's feelings, practicing self-care, cultivating mindfulness, and seeking support, mothers can cope with the physical discomfort and emotional stress that comes with breastfeeding difficulties.

Through self-compassion, mothers can build resilience, strength, and self-acceptance as they navigate through the challenges of motherhood and breastfeeding.

From Transforming Your Plugged Duct Experience From Discomfort to

Breastfeeding is a beautiful and natural experience that many mothers look forward to when they have a new baby. However, it is not always smooth sailing, and many mothers face challenges along the way.

One common issue that breastfeeding mothers may encounter is a plugged duct. This can be a painful and uncomfortable experience, but with the right knowledge and support, it can be overcome.

What is a Plugged Duct?

A plugged duct occurs when a milk duct in the breast becomes blocked, preventing milk from flowing freely. This can lead to a build-up of milk in the breast, causing pain, swelling, and inflammation.

Plugged ducts are common among breastfeeding mothers, especially in the early weeks after giving birth. They can be caused by a variety of factors, including improper latch, infrequent feedings, tight clothing, or pressure on the breast.

Symptoms of a Plugged Duct

If you are experiencing a plugged duct, you may notice the

following symptoms:

- A painful lump or area of hardness in the breast
- Redness and swelling in the affected area
- A feeling of fullness or heaviness in the breast
- Pain or tenderness when breastfeeding or touching the affected breast
- Flu-like symptoms, such as fever, chills, or body aches

It is important to address a plugged duct promptly to prevent it from developing into a more serious condition, such as mastitis, which is an infection of the breast tissue.

Tips for Preventing Plugged Ducts

While plugged ducts can occur for a variety of reasons, there are steps you can take to help prevent them from happening:

- Ensure a proper latch: A good latch is essential for effective breastfeeding and can help prevent plugged ducts. Make sure your baby is latched on correctly and seek help from a lactation consultant if needed.

- Nurse frequently: Breastfeeding frequently can help prevent milk from building up in the breast and reduce the risk of plugged ducts. Aim to nurse your baby on demand, at least every 2-3 hours.

- Empty the breast completely: Make sure to empty each breast fully during feedings to prevent milk from stagnating in the ducts. If your baby does not drain the breast completely, you can use a breast pump to express any remaining milk.

- Avoid tight clothing: Tight bras or clothing can put pressure on the breasts and impede milk flow. Opt for loose- fitting, comfortable clothing that allows for unrestricted movement.

- Use heat and massage: Applying heat to the affected breast and gently massaging the area can help loosen the blockage and promote milk flow. You can use a warm compress or take a warm shower before breastfeeding.

- Stay hydrated and eat well: Proper hydration and nutrition are important for maintaining a healthy milk supply and preventing plugged ducts. Drink plenty of water and eat a balanced diet rich in fruits, vegetables, and whole
grains.

Treatment for Plugged Ducts

If you develop a plugged duct, there are several steps you can take to help alleviate the discomfort and promote healing:

- Nurse frequently: Continuing to breastfeed on the affected side can help clear the blockage and reduce inflammation. Make sure to position your baby so that their chin points towards the affected area to help drain the duct.

- Apply heat: Using a warm compress or taking a warm shower

can help relax the muscles and improve blood flow to the affected breast. You can also try massaging the area gently while applying heat.

- Massage the affected area: Gently massaging the lump or area of hardness in a circular motion towards the nipple can help break up the blockage and promote milk flow. You can do this before or during breastfeeding.

- Change breastfeeding positions: Experimenting with different breastfeeding positions can help ensure that all areas of the breast are being drained effectively. Try the football hold, side-lying position, or laid-back breastfeeding.

- Take over-the-counter pain relievers: If you are experiencing pain or discomfort, you can take over-the-counter pain relievers such as ibuprofen or acetaminophen to help alleviate symptoms. Make sure to follow the recommended dosage.

- Rest and relax: Getting plenty of rest and relaxation can help your body heal and recover from a plugged duct. Try to avoid activities that put pressure on the affected breast and take breaks when needed.

- Seek support: If you are struggling with a plugged duct or breastfeeding in general, do not hesitate to reach out for help. Talk to a lactation consultant, your healthcare provider, or a breastfeeding support group for guidance and support.

Transforming Your Plugged Duct Experience

While dealing with a plugged duct can be a challenging and uncomfortable experience, it can also be an opportunity for growth and empowerment. By taking proactive steps to address the issue and seeking support when needed, you can transform your plugged duct experience into a positive and empowering one.

Chapter 10: The Path to Healing: Embracing Natural Remedies for Plugged Duct Relief

Breastfeeding is a beautiful and natural way to nourish your baby, but it can also come with its own set of challenges. One common issue that many breastfeeding mothers face is a plugged duct.

This painful condition occurs when a milk duct becomes blocked, leading to a buildup of milk and inflammation in the breast tissue.

Plugged ducts can be incredibly uncomfortable and can make breastfeeding difficult and painful. However, there are natural remedies that can help to alleviate the symptoms and promote healing. In this article, we will explore the path to healing plugged ducts through embracing natural remedies.

Understanding Plugged Ducts

Before we delve into natural remedies for plugged duct relief, it's important to understand what causes plugged ducts and how they can impact breastfeeding. Plugged ducts can occur for a variety of reasons, including:

- Infrequent or incomplete breastfeeding: If you are not

breastfeeding frequently enough or if your baby is not effectively draining your breasts during feedings, milk can back up and lead to a plugged duct.

- Pressure on the breast: Wearing tight clothing or using a poorly fitting bra can put pressure on the breast tissue, leading to blocked ducts.

- Poor latch: If your baby is not latching properly during feedings, it can prevent milk from flowing freely and increase the risk of plugged ducts.

- Stress or fatigue: Stress and fatigue can weaken the immune system and make you more susceptible to developing plugged ducts.

Symptoms of a plugged duct can include:

- A tender or painful lump in the breast
- Redness and swelling in the affected area
- A feeling of fullness or engorgement in the breast
- Warmth or heat emanating from the affected area
- Flu-like symptoms, such as fever and chills

If you suspect that you have a plugged duct, it's important to address it promptly to prevent it from developing into a more serious condition, such as mastitis. Mastitis is a painful infection of the breast tissue that can require medical intervention, so it's best to take steps to resolve a plugged duct as soon as possible.

Natural Remedies for Plugged Duct Relief

Fortunately, there are a variety of natural remedies that can help to alleviate the symptoms of a plugged duct and promote healing. Here are some effective natural remedies to consider:

1. Breastfeeding frequently: One of the best ways to prevent and treat plugged ducts is to breastfeed frequently and ensure that your baby is effectively draining your breasts during feedings. Try to nurse on demand and offer both breasts at each feeding to help prevent milk from backing up and causing blockages.

2. Warm compress: Applying a warm compress to the affected breast can help to promote milk flow and reduce inflammation. You can use a warm washcloth or a heating pad on a low setting to gently heat the breast before

feedings or pumping sessions.

3. Massage: Gently massaging the affected breast can help to break up the blockage and promote milk flow. You can use your fingers to massage the lump in a circular motion while breastfeeding or pumping to help release the trapped milk.

4. Lecithin supplements: Lecithin is a natural emulsifier that can help to prevent and treat plugged ducts by reducing the stickiness of breast milk. Taking lecithin supplements daily can help to promote healthy milk flow and prevent blockages from forming.

5. Cabbage leaves: Applying chilled cabbage leaves to the affected breast can help to reduce inflammation and discomfort associated with plugged ducts. Simply place a few cabbage leaves in the refrigerator until they are cold, then place them inside your bra against the affected breast for 20-30 minutes.

6. Epsom salt soak: Soaking your breasts in a warm bath with Epsom salt can help to reduce inflammation and promote healing of plugged ducts. Add a cup of Epsom salt to a warm bath and soak for 15-20 minutes, focusing on the affected breast.

7. Stay hydrated: Drinking plenty of water can help to thin out your breast milk and prevent it from becoming too thick and sticky, which can contribute to plugged ducts. Aim to drink at least 8-10 glasses of water per day to stay hydrated and support healthy milk production.

8. Rest and relaxation: Stress and fatigue can weaken the immune system and make you more susceptible to developing plugged ducts. Make sure to prioritize rest and relaxation, and ask for help with household chores and childcare to give yourself time to focus on healing.

9. Essential oils: Certain essential oils, such as lavender and chamomile, have anti-inflammatory and analgesic properties that can help to reduce pain and inflammation associated with plugged ducts. You can dilute a few drops of essential oil in a carrier oil, such as coconut or olive oil, and apply it to the affected breast for relief.

Nourishing Your Body, Nurturing Your Soul: Self-Care Practices for Plugged Ducts

Self-care is a vital aspect of maintaining overall health and well-being. It involves taking the time to nourish your body and nurture your soul, ensuring that you are in optimal condition to face life's challenges.

One common issue that many women face during their breastfeeding journey is plugged ducts. Plugged ducts can be painful and uncomfortable, but there are several self-care practices that can help alleviate the symptoms and promote healing.

What are Plugged Ducts?

Plugged ducts occur when milk ducts in the breast become blocked, preventing the flow of milk. This blockage can lead to a buildup of milk, causing pain, swelling, and inflammation in the affected area. Plugged ducts are a common issue for breastfeeding women, and they can be caused by a variety of factors, including:

- Infrequent or irregular breastfeeding or pumping
- Pressure on the breast from tight clothing or a poorly fitting bra
- Inadequate breast emptying
- Stress or fatigue

- Illness or infection

Symptoms of plugged ducts may include a tender, swollen lump in the breast, redness and warmth in the affected area, and a feeling of fullness or heaviness in the breast.

If left untreated, plugged ducts can lead to more serious complications, such as mastitis, a painful breast infection.

Self-Care Practices for Plugged Ducts

Fortunately, there are several self-care practices that can help relieve the symptoms of plugged ducts and promote healing.

These practices focus on nourishing your body and nurturing your soul, ensuring that you are taking care of yourself both physically and emotionally. Here are some self-care practices for plugged ducts that you can incorporate into your daily routine:

1. Breastfeed or Pump Frequently

One of the most effective ways to prevent and treat plugged ducts is to breastfeed or pump frequently. Regularly emptying your breasts helps to prevent milk from building up and causing blockages.

Aim to breastfeed or pump every 2-3 hours, or whenever your baby shows signs of hunger. If you are having trouble emptying your breasts, try massaging them gently while breastfeeding or pumping to help stimulate milk flow.

2. Apply Heat

Applying heat to the affected breast can help to relieve pain and inflammation caused by plugged ducts. You can use a warm compress, such as a warm washcloth or heating pad, to apply heat to the affected area.

Simply place the warm compress on the breast for 10-15 minutes at a time, several times a day. The heat can help to loosen the blockage and promote milk flow.

3. Massage the Breast

Massaging the affected breast can help to break up the blockage and promote milk flow. Gently massage the breast in a circular motion, starting at the outer edge and working your way towards the nipple. You can also try using a breast massage tool or your fingers to apply gentle pressure to the affected area. Massaging the breast can help to relieve pain and discomfort caused by plugged ducts.

4. Take a Warm Shower

Taking a warm shower can help to relax the muscles in the breast and promote milk flow. The warm water can help to soothe pain and inflammation caused by plugged ducts. While in the shower, gently massage the affected breast to help break up the blockage. You can also try expressing milk by hand while in the shower to help empty the breast.

5. Stay Hydrated

Staying hydrated is important for overall breast health and can help to prevent plugged ducts. Make sure to drink plenty of water throughout the day to keep your body hydrated and promote milk production. Aim to drink at least 8-10 glasses of water a day, or more if you are breastfeeding. Staying hydrated can help to keep your milk flowing smoothly and prevent blockages in the breast.

6. Get Plenty of Rest

Rest is essential for healing and recovery from plugged ducts. Make sure to get plenty of rest and take breaks throughout the day to relax and recharge.

Avoid overexerting yourself and listen to your body's signals. If you are feeling tired or run down, take a break and prioritize self-care. Getting enough rest can help to reduce stress and fatigue, which can contribute to plugged ducts.

7. Practice Self-Care

In addition to physical self-care practices, it is important to nurture your soul and take care of your emotional well-being. Practicing self-care can help to reduce stress and promote relaxation, which can aid in the healing process. Take time for yourself each day to do something that brings you joy and relaxation, such as reading a book, taking a walk, or practicing yoga. Prioritize self-care and make it a part of your daily routine.

8. Seek Support

If you are struggling with plugged ducts, don't be afraid to seek support from healthcare professionals or lactation consultants.

A Comprehensive Guide to Plugged Duct Relief: From Discomfort to Recovery

A plugged duct, also known as a clogged milk duct, is a common issue that many breastfeeding mothers face. It occurs when milk flow is blocked in a milk duct, leading to discomfort, pain, and potentially more serious complications if not addressed promptly.

In this comprehensive guide, we will explore the causes, symptoms, and treatment options for plugged ducts, as well as tips for prevention and recovery.

Causes of Plugged Ducts

Plugged ducts can be caused by a variety of factors, including:

1. Incomplete Emptying of the Breast: If the breast is not fully emptied during a feeding, milk can build up and block a duct.

2. Pressure on the Breast: Wearing tight clothing, using a poorly fitting bra, or sleeping in a position that puts pressure on the breast can also lead to plugged ducts.

3. Illness or Inflammation: Mastitis, a common breastfeeding-related infection, can cause inflammation in the breast tissue and block milk flow.

4. Stress: Stress can affect milk production and flow, leading to plugged ducts.

Symptoms of Plugged Ducts

The symptoms of a plugged duct can vary from mild to severe and may include:

1. A tender, painful lump in the breast
2. Redness and swelling in the affected area
3. A warm sensation in the breast
4. A decrease in milk supply from the affected breast
5. Flu-like symptoms, such as fever and chills

If you are experiencing any of these symptoms, it is important to seek treatment promptly to prevent the condition from worsening.

Treatment Options for Plugged Ducts

There are several treatment options available for plugged ducts, including:

1. Breastfeeding: Continuing to breastfeed from the affected breast can help to clear the blockage and reduce discomfort. Ensure that your baby is latching properly and feeding effectively to help empty the breast completely.

2. Warm Compress: Applying a warm compress to the affected breast before feeding can help to soften the blockage and

improve milk flow.

3. Massage: Gently massaging the affected area while feeding or pumping can help to break up the blockage and
promote milk flow.

4. Pumping: If your baby is having difficulty latching or if you are unable to breastfeed, pumping can help to empty the breast and relieve the blockage.

5. Rest and Hydration: Getting plenty of rest and staying hydrated can help to support your body's natural healing process and reduce the risk of developing further complications.

6. Over-the-Counter Pain Relief: If you are experiencing pain or discomfort, you may consider taking over-the- counter pain relief medication, such as ibuprofen, to help manage your symptoms.

Prevention of Plugged Ducts

While plugged ducts can be a common issue for breastfeeding mothers, there are steps you can take to help prevent them from occurring, including:

1. Ensure Proper Latch: Ensuring that your baby is latching properly can help to prevent milk from backing up in the ducts.

2. Empty the Breast Completely: Make sure to empty each breast completely during feedings to prevent milk from building

up and causing blockages.

3. Avoid Tight Clothing: Wearing loose-fitting clothing and bras can help to prevent pressure on the breasts and reduce the risk of plugged ducts.

4. Manage Stress: Finding ways to manage stress, such as practicing relaxation techniques or seeking support from a lactation consultant, can help to support milk production and flow.

5. Maintain Good Hygiene: Keeping the breast and nipple area clean and dry can help to prevent infections that can lead to inflammation and blocked ducts.

Recovery from Plugged Ducts

With prompt treatment and proper care, most plugged ducts can be resolved within a few days. However, if you are experiencing persistent symptoms or if the condition worsens, it is important to seek medical attention to rule out more serious complications, such as mastitis.

In addition to the treatment options mentioned above, there are a few additional tips that can help to promote recovery from plugged ducts, including:

1. Continue to Breastfeed: Continuing to breastfeed from the affected breast can help to clear the blockage and promote healing.

2. Use Cold Compresses: Applying a cold compress to the affected breast after feeding can help to reduce inflammation and alleviate pain.

3. Take Warm Showers: Taking warm showers can help to relax the breast tissue and promote milk flow.

1. Practice Good Breastfeeding Positions: Finding comfortable and effective breastfeeding positions can help to ensure proper milk flow and prevent future blockages.

2. Seek Support: If you are struggling with plugged ducts or other breastfeeding challenges, don't hesitate to seek support from a lactation consultant, healthcare provider, or breastfeeding support group.

Chapter 11: Healing from Within: Natural Remedies and Self-Care Practices for Plugged Ducts Healing from Within

Plugged ducts are a common issue that many breastfeeding mothers face. They occur when milk ducts become blocked, leading to pain, swelling, and sometimes infection.

While plugged ducts can be uncomfortable and frustrating, there are several natural remedies and self-care practices that can help to alleviate symptoms and promote healing from within.

In this article, we will explore the causes and symptoms of plugged ducts, as well as various natural remedies and self-care practices that can help to prevent and treat this common breastfeeding issue.

By taking a holistic approach to healing from within, breastfeeding mothers can find relief from plugged ducts and continue to provide their babies with the nourishment they need.

Causes and Symptoms of Plugged Ducts

Plugged ducts can occur for a variety of reasons, including:

- Poor latching or positioning during breastfeeding
- Infrequent or irregular nursing sessions
- Pressure on the breasts from tight clothing or a poorly fitting bra
- Stress or fatigue
- Dehydration
- Mastitis (an infection of the breast tissue)

The symptoms of plugged ducts can vary, but common signs include:

- A hard, tender lump in the breast
- Redness or swelling in the affected area
- Pain or discomfort while breastfeeding
- Fever or flu-like symptoms (if an infection is present)

If left untreated, plugged ducts can lead to more serious complications, such as mastitis or abscess formation. It is important for breastfeeding mothers to address plugged ducts promptly to prevent these issues and promote healing from within.

Natural Remedies for Plugged Ducts

There are several natural remedies that can help to alleviate symptoms of plugged ducts and promote healing from within. Some common remedies include:

- Warm compress: Applying a warm compress to the affected breast can help to reduce pain and swelling, and encourage milk flow. Simply soak a washcloth in warm water and place it on the breast for 10-15 minutes several times a day.

- Massage: Gently massaging the affected breast can help to break up the blockage and promote milk flow. Use circular motions and gentle pressure to massage the lump, moving towards the nipple.

- Nursing: Continuing to breastfeed regularly can help to prevent and treat plugged ducts. Make sure your baby is latching properly and emptying the breast completely during each feeding.

- Pumping: If your baby is having trouble nursing from the affected breast, pumping can help to empty the breast and relieve the blockage. Use a breast pump on a low setting to avoid causing further irritation.

- Rest and hydration: Getting plenty of rest and staying hydrated are important for promoting healing from within. Make sure to drink plenty of water and take breaks when needed to avoid overexertion.

Self-Care Practices for Plugged Ducts

In addition to natural remedies, there are several self-care practices that can help to prevent and treat plugged ducts. Some self-care practices to consider include:

- Proper nutrition: Eating a balanced diet rich in fruits, vegetables, and whole grains can help to support overall health and promote healing from within. Avoiding excessive caffeine and alcohol can also help to prevent plugged ducts.

- Stress management: Stress can contribute to blocked ducts, so finding ways to manage stress is important for healing from within. Practice relaxation techniques such as deep breathing, meditation, or yoga to help reduce stress levels.

- Gentle exercise: Engaging in gentle exercise, such as walking or swimming, can help to improve circulation and promote healing from within. Avoid high-impact activities that may put pressure on the breasts.

- Supportive clothing: Wearing a well-fitting bra that provides proper support can help to prevent plugged ducts. Avoid tight bras or underwire bras that may constrict milk flow.

- Consult a lactation consultant: If you are experiencing frequent plugged ducts or having trouble breastfeeding, consider consulting a lactation consultant for guidance and support. They can help you address any underlying issues and develop a plan for healing from within.

By incorporating natural remedies and self-care practices into your routine, you can promote healing from within and find relief from plugged ducts. Remember to listen to your body, rest when needed, and seek support from healthcare providers or lactation consultants as needed.

Healing from within is a holistic approach to treating plugged ducts that focuses on natural remedies and self- care practices.

By addressing the underlying causes of plugged ducts and promoting healing from within, breastfeeding mothers can find relief from this common issue and continue to provide their babies with the nourishment they need.

If you are experiencing symptoms of plugged ducts, consider incorporating natural remedies such as warm compresses, massage, and proper nutrition into your routine.

Additionally, practicing self-care techniques such as stress management, gentle exercise, and supportive clothing can help to prevent and treat plugged ducts.

The Journey to Relief: Strategies for Overcoming Plugged Duct Challenges

Breastfeeding is a beautiful and natural process that provides numerous benefits to both the mother and the baby. However, it can also come with its own set of challenges, one of which is plugged ducts.

Plugged ducts occur when a milk duct in the breast becomes blocked, causing milk to back up and create a painful lump.

This can be a frustrating and uncomfortable experience for breastfeeding mothers, but there are strategies that can help overcome plugged duct challenges and provide relief.

Understanding the Causes of Plugged Ducts

Plugged ducts can be caused by a variety of factors, including:

- Infrequent or irregular breastfeeding or pumping: When milk is not regularly and completely emptied from the breast, it can lead to a buildup of milk and the formation of a plugged duct.

- Pressure on the breast: Wearing tight clothing or bras, carrying heavy bags on the shoulder, or sleeping in a position that puts pressure on the breast can also contribute to the development of plugged ducts.
- Poor latch: If the baby is not latching properly during breastfeeding, it can prevent the breast from being fully emptied

and increase the risk of plugged ducts.

- Stress and fatigue: Stress and fatigue can weaken the immune system and make it more difficult for the body to fight off infections, including those that can lead to plugged ducts.

Recognizing the Symptoms of Plugged Ducts

It is important for breastfeeding mothers to be able to recognize the symptoms of plugged ducts so that they can take action to address the issue promptly. Some common symptoms of plugged ducts include:

- A painful lump or area of hardness in the breast
- Redness and swelling in the affected area
- Warmth and tenderness to the touch
- A feeling of fullness or engorgement in the breast
- Flu-like symptoms, such as fever and chills

If you are experiencing any of these symptoms, it is important to seek help from a healthcare provider or lactation consultant to determine the best course of action for relieving the plugged duct.

Strategies for Overcoming Plugged Duct Challenges

There are several strategies that can help breastfeeding mothers overcome plugged duct challenges and find relief. These strategies include:

1. Nursing or Pumping Frequently

One of the most effective ways to prevent and treat plugged ducts is to nurse or pump frequently. This helps to ensure that the breast is fully emptied of milk and reduces the risk of milk buildup and blockages. If you are experiencing a plugged duct, nursing or pumping more frequently can help to clear the blockage and provide relief.

2. Using Warm Compresses

Applying a warm compress to the affected breast can help to reduce pain and inflammation associated with plugged ducts. A warm shower or warm washcloth can be used to gently massage the breast and encourage milk flow. Some mothers find relief by using a warm rice sock or gel pad on the affected area.

3. Massaging the Breast

Gentle breast massage can help to break up the blockage and promote milk flow. Using circular motions and gentle pressure, massage the affected breast towards the nipple to help release the plugged duct. You can also try massaging the breast while nursing or pumping to help clear the blockage.

4. Changing Nursing Positions

Changing nursing positions can help to ensure that the breast is fully emptied during breastfeeding. Experiment with different positions, such as the football hold or side-lying position, to find a comfortable and effective way to nurse your baby. This can help to prevent plugged ducts from occurring and provide relief if you are already experiencing a blockage.

5. Ensuring Proper Latch

Ensuring that your baby has a proper latch during breastfeeding is essential for preventing plugged ducts. A poor latch can prevent the breast from being fully emptied and increase the risk of milk buildup and blockages. If you are having trouble with your baby's latch, seek help from a lactation consultant or healthcare provider to address the issue.

6. Rest and Self-Care

Rest and self-care are important for overall health and well-being, especially when dealing with plugged ducts. Make sure to get plenty of rest, stay hydrated, and eat a healthy diet to support your body's ability to fight off infections and heal. Taking time for yourself and practicing self-care activities, such as gentle exercise, meditation, or relaxation techniques, can also help to reduce stress and promote healing.

7. Seeking Support

Dealing with plugged ducts can be a challenging and frustrating experience, but you are not alone. Reach out to a healthcare provider, lactation consultant, or breastfeeding support group for help and guidance. Talking to other breastfeeding mothers who have experienced plugged ducts can provide valuable insights and support as you work to overcome this common challenge.

8. Using Natural Remedies

There are several natural remedies that can help to relieve plugged ducts and promote healing.

Embracing Wellness: A Holistic Approach to Plugged Duct Relief Embracing Wellness

Breastfeeding is a beautiful and natural process that provides numerous benefits to both mother and baby. However, it can also come with its challenges, one of which is plugged ducts.

A plugged duct occurs when a milk duct in the breast becomes blocked, leading to pain, swelling, and sometimes infection. While plugged ducts are common and usually resolve on their own, they can be incredibly uncomfortable and disruptive to the breastfeeding relationship.

In this article, we will explore a holistic approach to plugged duct relief, focusing on the importance of embracing wellness in all aspects of your life. By taking a comprehensive and proactive approach to your health and well-being, you can not only find relief from plugged ducts but also promote overall wellness and vitality.

Understanding Plugged Ducts

Before we delve into holistic approaches to plugged duct relief, it's important to understand what causes plugged ducts and how they can be identified. Plugged ducts typically occur when milk is not effectively removed from the breast, leading to a build-up of milk in the duct. This can happen for a variety of reasons, including:

- Poor latch or positioning during breastfeeding
- Infrequent or incomplete emptying of the breast
- Pressure on the breast from tight clothing or a poorly fitting bra
- Stress or fatigue, which can affect milk flow
  - Hormonal changes, such as during menstruation or weaning

Symptoms of a plugged duct can include:

- A tender or painful lump in the breast
- Redness or swelling in a localized area
- A feeling of fullness or heaviness in the breast
- Pain or discomfort while breastfeeding or pumping
- Flu-like symptoms, such as fever or chills

If you suspect you have a plugged duct, it's important to address it promptly to prevent further complications, such as mastitis. In most cases, plugged ducts can be resolved with a combination of self-care measures and gentle interventions.

Embracing Wellness: A Holistic Approach

When it comes to addressing plugged ducts, taking a holistic approach that considers the whole person is key. Holistic wellness focuses on the interconnectedness of mind, body, and spirit, recognizing that each aspect of our being influences the others. By embracing wellness in all areas of your life, you can support your body's natural healing processes and promote overall health and vitality.

Here are some holistic approaches to plugged duct relief that you may find helpful:

1. Nurture Your Body

One of the most important aspects of holistic wellness is nurturing your body with nourishing foods, plenty of water, and adequate rest. Eating a balanced diet rich in fruits, vegetables, whole grains, and lean proteins can provide your body with the nutrients it needs to function optimally. Staying hydrated by drinking plenty of water can help to keep your milk flowing and prevent dehydration, which can contribute to plugged ducts. Getting enough rest and prioritizing self-care can also support your body's ability to heal and recover.

In addition to nourishing your body with healthy foods and rest, you may also consider incorporating supportive herbs and supplements into your routine. For example, lecithin is a supplement that has been shown to help prevent plugged ducts by reducing the stickiness of breast milk. Other herbs, such as fenugreek, blessed thistle, and fennel, may also support milk production and flow.

2. Practice Gentle Breast Massage and Compression

When you have a plugged duct, gentle massage and compression can help to break up the blockage and promote milk flow. Before breastfeeding or pumping, warm your breast with a warm compress or shower to help soften the blockage.

Then, using gentle circular motions, massage the affected area towards the nipple to encourage the milk to flow. You can also try applying gentle pressure to the blocked duct with your fingers or a warm compress to help release the blockage.

In addition to massage and compression, you may also find relief from using a warm compress or heating pad on the affected breast.

 The heat can help to reduce pain and swelling, as well as promote milk flow. Just be sure to use a gentle heat source and avoid applying excessive pressure or heat to the breast, as this can cause further irritation.

3. Maintain Good Breastfeeding Practices

Proper breastfeeding techniques are essential for preventing and relieving plugged ducts. Ensuring a good latch and positioning during breastfeeding can help to ensure that your baby is effectively removing milk from the breast.

If you are experiencing pain or discomfort while breastfeeding, it's important to seek support from a lactation consultant or breastfeeding counselor to address any issues that may be contributing to plugged ducts.

In addition to proper latch and positioning, it's important to breastfeed frequently and thoroughly to prevent plugged ducts. Aim to breastfeed on demand, offering your baby the breast whenever   they   show   hunger   cues.

Chapter 12: The Power of Self-Healing: Finding Relief from Plugged Ducts Naturally

Breastfeeding is a beautiful and natural experience that provides numerous benefits for both mother and baby. However, it is not without its challenges.

One common issue that many breastfeeding mothers face is plugged ducts. Plugged ducts occur when milk flow is blocked in the ducts of the breast, causing pain, swelling, and even infection.

Plugged ducts can be incredibly painful and frustrating for breastfeeding mothers. They can make it difficult to nurse, leading to decreased milk supply and potential complications such as mastitis. While plugged ducts are a common issue, there are ways to find relief and promote healing naturally.

The power of self-healing is a concept that emphasizes the body's ability to heal itself with the right support and resources. When it comes to plugged ducts, there are several natural remedies and techniques that can help to alleviate symptoms and promote healing.

One of the most effective ways to find relief from plugged ducts naturally is through frequent nursing or pumping. By emptying the breast regularly, you can help to clear the blockage and prevent further buildup of milk. It is important to nurse on demand and ensure that both breasts are fully emptied during each feeding session.

In addition to frequent nursing, applying heat to the affected breast can help to alleviate pain and promote healing. Warm compresses, hot showers, or a heating pad can all be effective in reducing inflammation and improving milk flow.

Gentle massage of the affected breast can also help to break up the blockage and encourage milk flow.

Another natural remedy for plugged ducts is to ensure proper hydration and nutrition. Drinking plenty of water and eating a balanced diet rich in fruits, vegetables, and whole grains can help to support overall breast health and prevent future blockages.

Avoiding tight clothing or bras that constrict the breasts can also help to prevent plugged ducts from occurring.

Herbal remedies can also be effective in promoting healing from plugged ducts. Lecithin supplements, which are derived from soybeans, can help to prevent blockages by reducing the stickiness of breast milk. Other herbs such as fenugreek, blessed thistle, and dandelion root can also help to support milk production and flow.

In addition to these natural remedies, self-care practices such as rest, relaxation, and stress management can also play a role in promoting healing from plugged ducts. Taking time to rest and care for yourself can help to reduce inflammation and support the body's natural healing process.

It is important to remember that plugged ducts can be a sign of an underlying issue, such as improper latch, positioning, or milk supply. If you are experiencing recurrent plugged ducts or severe symptoms, it is important to seek support from a lactation consultant or healthcare provider.

In conclusion, finding relief from plugged ducts naturally is possible through a combination of self-care practices, natural remedies, and support.

By nurturing your body and providing it with the resources it needs to heal, you can overcome the challenges of plugged ducts and continue to enjoy the many benefits of breastfeeding. Trust in the power of self-healing and give your body the care and attention it deserves.

Transforming Discomfort into Ease

Breastfeeding is a beautiful and natural way to nourish your baby, but it can also come with its fair share of challenges. One common issue that many breastfeeding mothers face is plugged ducts.

Plugged ducts can be painful and uncomfortable, but with the right strategies and techniques, you can transform that discomfort into ease.

In this guide, we will explore what plugged ducts are, why they occur, and most importantly, how you can find relief and prevent them from happening in the future.

By understanding the causes of plugged ducts and implementing the right strategies, you can make your breastfeeding journey a more comfortable and enjoyable experience for both you and your baby.

What are Plugged Ducts?

Plugged ducts occur when a milk duct in the breast becomes blocked, preventing the flow of milk. This blockage can cause the milk to back up and create a painful lump in the breast. Plugged ducts are a common issue for breastfeeding mothers, and they can be caused by a variety of factors, including:

- Infrequent or irregular nursing or pumping

- Pressure on the breast from tight clothing or a poorly fitting bra
- Improper latch or positioning during breastfeeding
- Stress or fatigue
- Dehydration
- Illness or infection

Symptoms of plugged ducts can include:

- A painful lump or area of hardness in the breast
- Redness or warmth in the affected area
- Swelling or tenderness
- A decrease in milk supply from the affected breast

If left untreated, plugged ducts can lead to more serious issues such as mastitis, a painful and potentially dangerous breast infection. It is important to address plugged ducts promptly to prevent further complications and find relief from the discomfort.

Finding Relief from Plugged Ducts

If you are experiencing plugged ducts, there are several strategies you can try to find relief and promote milk flow. Here are some tips to help you transform discomfort into ease:

1. Nurse or Pump Frequently: One of the most effective ways to clear a plugged duct is to nurse or pump frequently. Emptying the breast regularly can help to relieve the blockage and promote milk flow. Try nursing on the affected side first, and switch positions frequently to ensure that all areas of the

breast are being drained.

2. Apply Heat: Applying heat to the affected breast can help to reduce pain and inflammation and promote milk flow. You can use a warm compress, a heating pad, or take a warm shower to help loosen the blockage. Gently massaging the affected area while applying heat can also be helpful.

3. Massage the Breast: Massaging the affected breast can help to break up the blockage and promote milk flow. Use gentle circular motions with your fingertips to massage the lump in the direction of the nipple. You can also try hand expressing or using a breast pump to help clear the duct.

4. Practice Good Breastfeeding Hygiene: Make sure to keep your breasts clean and dry to prevent infection and further complications. Wear loose-fitting clothing and a well-fitting bra to avoid putting pressure on the breasts. Change nursing pads frequently and wash your hands before each feeding or pumping session.

5. Stay Hydrated and Well-Nourished: Drinking plenty of water and eating a balanced diet can help to support milk production and prevent plugged ducts. Make sure to stay hydrated throughout the day and eat foods rich in nutrients such as protein, vitamins, and minerals.

6. Get Plenty of Rest: Rest and relaxation are important for maintaining a healthy milk supply and preventing plugged ducts.

Make time to rest and recharge, and ask for help from family and friends if needed. Stress and fatigue can contribute to the development of plugged ducts, so it is important to take care of yourself.

7. Seek Support: If you are struggling with plugged ducts or other breastfeeding challenges, don't hesitate to reach out for support.

Talk to a lactation consultant, your healthcare provider, or other breastfeeding mothers for guidance and encouragement. You are not alone, and there are resources available to help you navigate this journey.

Preventing Plugged Ducts

While plugged ducts can be a common issue for breastfeeding mothers, there are steps you can take to prevent them from occurring in the future. Here are some tips for preventing plugged ducts and maintaining a healthy breastfeeding relationship:

1. Nurse on Demand: Nursing on demand can help to prevent engorgement and ensure that your breasts are being emptied regularly.

2. Try to nurse your baby whenever they show signs of hunger, rather than on a strict schedule. This can help to prevent milk from backing up and causing blockages.

Ensure Proper Latch and Positioning: A proper latch and positioning are essential for effective breastfeeding and can help to prevent plugged ducts.

3. Make sure that your baby is latching correctly and that they are positioned comfortably at the breast.

Mindful Living with Plugged Ducts: Embracing Self-Care for Healing

In today's fast-paced world, it can be easy to get caught up in the hustle and bustle of daily life. From work deadlines to family obligations, it can feel like there is always something demanding our attention.

In the midst of all this chaos, it is important to remember to take care of ourselves and practice mindfulness in order to maintain our overall well-being.

One common issue that many women face during their breastfeeding journey is plugged ducts. Plugged ducts occur when a milk duct in the breast becomes blocked, causing milk to back up and create a painful lump.

This can be a frustrating and uncomfortable experience, but with the right approach, it can be managed effectively.

Mindful living is a practice that involves being present in the moment, paying attention to our thoughts and feelings without judgment, and taking care of ourselves both physically and emotionally.

When it comes to dealing with plugged ducts, embracing self-care and mindfulness can be incredibly beneficial in promoting healing and preventing future issues.

One of the first steps in practicing mindful living with plugged ducts is to listen to your body and pay attention to any signs of discomfort.

If you notice a painful lump in your breast or experience any other symptoms of a plugged duct, it is important to address it promptly. Ignoring the issue can lead to more serious complications, such as mastitis, which is an infection of the breast tissue.

When dealing with a plugged duct, self-care is key. This includes staying well-hydrated, getting plenty of rest, and eating a healthy diet. It is also important to continue breastfeeding or pumping regularly to help clear the blockage.

Applying warm compresses to the affected breast and gently massaging the area can also help to loosen the blockage and promote milk flow.

In addition to physical self-care, it is important to take care of your emotional well-being as well. Dealing with a plugged duct can be stressful and overwhelming, so it is important to practice self-compassion and be gentle with yourself. Remember that it is not your fault and that these issues are common among breastfeeding women.

Mindfulness can also be a powerful tool in managing the stress and anxiety that can come with dealing with plugged ducts. By practicing mindfulness techniques such as deep breathing, meditation, and yoga, you can help to calm your mind and reduce your overall stress levels. This can not only help to promote healing but can also prevent future issues from arising.

Another important aspect of mindful living with plugged ducts is seeking support from others.

Whether it is talking to a lactation consultant, joining a breastfeeding support group, or reaching out to friends and family for help, having a strong support system can make a world of difference.

Being able to share your struggles and receive encouragement from others can help to alleviate feelings of isolation and provide you with the strength and motivation to keep going.

It is also important to remember that self-care is not selfish. Taking the time to care for yourself and prioritize your well-being is essential in order to be able to care for others effectively. By practicing self-care and mindfulness, you are not only benefiting yourself but also those around you.

In conclusion, mindful living with plugged ducts involves embracing self-care and practicing mindfulness in order to promote healing and overall well-being. By listening to your body, taking care of yourself both physically and emotionally, seeking support from others, and practicing mindfulness techniques, you can effectively manage plugged ducts and prevent future issues from arising.

Remember that self-care is not selfish, and by prioritizing your own well-being, you are better able to care for those around you. Embrace self-care, practice mindfulness, and remember to be gentle with yourself during this challenging time.

Chapter 13: The Road to Recovery: Strategies for Clearing Plugged Ducts and Finding Relief The Road to Recovery

Breastfeeding is a beautiful and natural process that provides numerous benefits for both mother and baby. However, it can also come with its own set of challenges, one of which is plugged ducts.

 Plugged ducts occur when milk is not effectively removed from the breast, leading to a blockage in the milk duct. This can be painful and uncomfortable for the mother, and can also impact milk supply and overall breastfeeding success.

If you are experiencing a plugged duct, it's important to take action quickly to clear the blockage and find relief. In this article, we will discuss the road to recovery for plugged ducts, including strategies for clearing the blockage and finding relief.

Signs and Symptoms of Plugged Ducts

Plugged ducts can be uncomfortable and painful, and it's important to recognize the signs and symptoms so that you can take action quickly. Some common signs of plugged ducts include:

- A tender or painful lump in the breast
- Redness or swelling in the affected area
- A feeling of fullness or heaviness in the breast
- Pain or discomfort while breastfeeding or pumping
- Flu-like symptoms, such as fever or chills

If you are experiencing any of these symptoms, it's important to address the issue promptly to prevent further complications.

Strategies for Clearing Plugged Ducts

There are several strategies that can help to clear plugged ducts and provide relief. Here are some effective methods to consider:

1. Nurse or Pump Frequently: One of the most important things you can do to clear a plugged duct is to nurse or pump frequently.

2. This helps to keep the milk flowing and prevent further blockages from forming. Make sure to empty the affected breast completely during each feeding or pumping session.

3. Apply Heat: Applying heat to the affected breast can help to relieve pain and discomfort, as well as encourage milk flow. You can use a warm compress, a heating pad, or take a warm shower to help loosen the blockage.

4. Massage the Breast: Gently massaging the affected breast can help to break up the blockage and promote milk flow. You can use circular motions or gentle pressure to massage the breast while nursing or pumping.

5. Change Nursing Positions: Changing nursing positions can help to ensure that all areas of the breast are effectively drained. Experiment with different positions, such as the football hold or side-lying position, to find the most comfortable and effective option for you.

6. Use a Breast Pump: If nursing alone is not effective in clearing the blockage, you can also use a breast pump

to help empty the affected breast. Make sure to use the pump on a low setting to avoid causing further discomfort.

7. Stay Hydrated and Rest: It's important to stay hydrated and get plenty of rest while dealing with a plugged duct. Drink plenty of water and take breaks to rest and relax throughout the day.

8. Take Over-the-Counter Pain Medication: If you are experiencing pain or discomfort, you can take over-the- counter pain medication, such as ibuprofen or acetaminophen, to help alleviate symptoms.

9. Consult a Lactation Consultant: If you are struggling to clear a plugged duct or experiencing persistent symptoms, it's important to consult a lactation consultant for guidance and support. They can provide personalized advice and strategies to

help you find relief.

Finding Relief and Preventing Future Plugged Ducts

In addition to clearing a plugged duct, it's important to take steps to prevent future blockages from occurring. Here are some strategies to help you find relief and prevent plugged ducts in the future:

1. Maintain Good Breastfeeding Practices: Ensuring that your baby is latching correctly and effectively draining the breast during feedings can help to prevent plugged ducts. Make sure to nurse frequently and empty the breast completely during each feeding.

2. Avoid Tight Clothing: Wearing tight clothing or bras can put pressure on the breasts and lead to blocked ducts. Opt for loose-fitting, comfortable clothing and bras that provide adequate support.

3. Practice Good Hygiene: Keeping the breast and nipple area clean and dry can help to prevent infections and blockages. Make sure to wash your hands before breastfeeding and use gentle cleansers to clean the breast.

4. Manage Stress: Stress can impact milk supply and breastfeeding success, so it's important to manage stress levels and prioritize self-care. Practice relaxation techniques, such as deep breathing or meditation, to help reduce stress.

5. Stay Active: Regular physical activity can help to improve circulation and promote milk flow. Incorporate gentle exercise, such as walking or yoga, into your daily routine to help prevent plugged ducts.

Use Warm Compresses: Applying warm compresses to the breast before nursing or pumping can help to stimulate milk flow and prevent blockages.

Chapter: Natural Remedies and Self-Care Practices for Plugged Ducts

Breastfeeding is a beautiful and natural way to nourish your baby, but it can also come with its challenges. One common issue that many breastfeeding mothers face is plugged ducts.

A plugged duct occurs when a milk duct in the breast becomes blocked, causing milk to back up and create a painful lump. This can be a frustrating and uncomfortable experience, but there are natural remedies and self-care practices that can help you find balance and comfort while dealing with plugged ducts.

Understanding Plugged Ducts

Plugged ducts can occur for a variety of reasons, including:

- Infrequent or irregular nursing or pumping
- Pressure on the breast from tight clothing or a poorly fitting bra
- Stress or fatigue
- Poor latch or positioning while breastfeeding
- Dehydration or poor nutrition

When a milk duct becomes blocked, it can cause pain, swelling, and tenderness in the affected breast. You may also notice a hard lump or redness on the surface of the breast. If left untreated, a plugged duct can lead to mastitis, a more serious condition that causes inflammation and infection in the breast tissue.

Natural Remedies for Plugged Ducts

If you are experiencing a plugged duct, there are several natural remedies that can help alleviate your symptoms and promote healing. Some of these remedies include:

1. Warm Compress: Applying a warm compress to the affected breast can help to relieve pain and swelling, as well as encourage milk flow. You can use a warm washcloth or a heating pad on a low setting for 10-15 minutes several times a day.

2. Massage: Gently massaging the affected breast can help to break up the blockage and improve milk flow. You can use your fingers or a breast massage tool to massage the area in a circular motion towards the nipple.

3. Nursing or Pumping: Nursing or pumping frequently can help to clear the blockage and prevent it from recurring. Make sure to empty the affected breast completely during each feeding or pumping session.

4. Rest and Hydration: Getting plenty of rest and staying hydrated can help to support your body's natural healing process. Make sure to drink plenty of water and eat a nutritious diet to promote overall health.

5. Herbal Remedies: Some herbs, such as fenugreek and blessed thistle, are known for their lactation-boosting properties

and can help to improve milk flow. You can take these herbs in supplement form or drink them as a tea.

Self-Care Practices for Plugged Ducts

In addition to natural remedies, there are several self-care practices that can help you find balance and comfort while dealing with plugged ducts. Some of these practices include:

1. Proper Latch and Positioning: Ensuring that your baby has a proper latch and positioning while breastfeeding can help to prevent plugged ducts from occurring. Make sure that your baby is latched on correctly and that their nose is aligned with your nipple.

2. Stress Management: Managing stress and finding ways to relax can help to prevent plugged ducts and promote healing. You can try practices such as deep breathing, meditation, yoga, or mindfulness to reduce stress levels.

3. Gentle Exercise: Engaging in gentle exercise, such as walking or swimming, can help to improve circulation and promote healing in the affected breast. Make sure to wear a supportive bra and avoid high-impact activities that may exacerbate your symptoms.

4. Supportive Clothing: Wearing a supportive and properly fitting bra can help to reduce pressure on the breast and prevent plugged ducts from occurring. Make sure to choose a bra that provides adequate support and does not constrict the breast tissue.

5. Cold Compress: In addition to warm compresses, applying a cold compress to the affected breast can help to reduce pain and swelling. You can use a cold pack or a bag of frozen vegetables wrapped in a towel for 10-15 minutes at a time.

Finding Balance and Comfort

Dealing with plugged ducts can be a challenging and uncomfortable experience, but with the right natural remedies and self-care practices, you can find balance and comfort while promoting healing in your breast. It is important to listen to your body and seek support from a lactation consultant or healthcare provider if you are experiencing persistent symptoms or complications.

Remember to prioritize self-care and take time to rest and relax during this time. Breastfeeding is a beautiful and natural bonding experience between you and your baby, and by taking care of yourself, you can continue to provide the best possible nourishment for your little one. Stay hydrated, eat nutritious foods, and practice gentle exercise to support your body's healing process.

In conclusion, finding balance and comfort while dealing with plugged ducts is possible with natural remedies and self-care practices.

The Healing Journey: Navigating Plugged Ducts with Grace and Resilience

Breastfeeding is a beautiful and natural process that can provide numerous benefits for both mother and baby. However, it is not always smooth sailing, and many women may encounter challenges along the way.

One common issue that breastfeeding mothers may face is plugged ducts. Plugged ducts can be painful and uncomfortable, but with the right knowledge and support, they can be successfully navigated with grace and resilience.

What are Plugged Ducts?

Plugged ducts occur when milk is not properly drained from the breast, leading to a blockage in one of the milk ducts. This blockage can cause the affected area of the breast to become swollen, tender, and painful to the touch.

Plugged ducts can also cause a decrease in milk supply and can lead to more serious issues such as mastitis if not addressed promptly.

Plugged ducts can be caused by a variety of factors, including:

- Infrequent or incomplete emptying of the breast
- Pressure on the breast from tight clothing or a poorly fitting bra

- Poor latch or positioning during breastfeeding
- Stress or fatigue
- Dehydration
    - A sudden increase in milk supply Symptoms of Plugged Ducts

The symptoms of plugged ducts can vary from woman to woman, but common signs include:

- A tender, painful lump in the breast
- Redness and swelling in the affected area
- A feeling of fullness or heaviness in the breast
- Pain or discomfort while nursing
- A low-grade fever or flu-like symptoms

It is important to note that not all lumps in the breast are plugged ducts, and any persistent lumps or changes in the breast should be evaluated by a healthcare provider.

Navigating Plugged Ducts with Grace and Resilience

Dealing with plugged ducts can be challenging, but with the right mindset and support, it is possible to navigate this common breastfeeding issue with grace and resilience. Here are some tips to help you through the healing journey of plugged ducts:

1. Keep Nursing

One of the most important things you can do when dealing with plugged ducts is to continue nursing your baby. Nursing frequently and ensuring that the affected breast is fully drained can help to clear the blockage and

In addition to natural remedies, there are several self-care practices that can help you find balance and comfort while dealing with plugged ducts. Some of these practices include:

6. Proper Latch and Positioning: Ensuring that your baby has a proper latch and positioning while breastfeeding can help to prevent plugged ducts from occurring. Make sure that your baby is latched on correctly and that their nose is aligned with your nipple.

7. Stress Management: Managing stress and finding ways to relax can help to prevent plugged ducts and promote healing. You can try practices such as deep breathing, meditation, yoga, or mindfulness to reduce stress levels.

8. Gentle Exercise: Engaging in gentle exercise, such as walking or swimming, can help to improve circulation and promote healing in the affected breast. Make sure to wear a supportive bra and avoid high-impact activities that may exacerbate your symptoms.

9. Supportive Clothing: Wearing a supportive and properly fitting bra can help to reduce pressure on the breast and prevent plugged ducts from occurring. Make sure to choose a bra that provides adequate support and does not constrict the breast tissue.

10. Cold Compress: In addition to warm compresses, applying a cold compress to the affected breast can help to reduce pain and

swelling. You can use a cold pack or a bag of frozen vegetables wrapped in a towel for 10-15 minutes at a time.

Finding Balance and Comfort

Dealing with plugged ducts can be a challenging and uncomfortable experience, but with the right natural remedies and self-care practices, you can find balance and comfort while promoting healing in your breast.

It is important to listen to your body and seek support from a lactation consultant or healthcare provider if you are experiencing persistent symptoms or complications.

Remember to prioritize self-care and take time to rest and relax during this time. Breastfeeding is a beautiful and natural bonding experience between you and your baby, and by taking care of yourself, you can continue to provide the best possible nourishment for your little one. Stay hydrated, eat nutritious foods, and practice gentle exercise to support your body's healing process.

In conclusion, finding balance and comfort while dealing with plugged ducts is possible with natural remedies and self-care practices.

Chapter 14: Empowering Yourself with Knowledge

Breastfeeding is a beautiful and natural way to nourish your baby, but it can also come with its challenges. One common issue that many breastfeeding mothers face is plugged ducts.

A plugged duct occurs when a milk duct in the breast becomes blocked, causing milk to back up and create a painful lump.

This can be a frustrating and uncomfortable experience, but with the right knowledge and techniques, you can effectively relieve plugged ducts and continue to breastfeed successfully.

In this comprehensive guide, we will explore the causes and symptoms of plugged ducts, as well as provide you with a variety of strategies for relieving them.

By empowering yourself with knowledge and understanding, you can confidently navigate this common breastfeeding obstacle and ensure a positive breastfeeding experience for both you and your baby.

Causes of Plugged Ducts

Plugged ducts can occur for a variety of reasons, but they are most commonly caused by a buildup of milk in the ducts. This can happen for several reasons, including:

- Poor milk drainage: If milk is not effectively removed from the breast, it can accumulate and block the ducts. This can happen if your baby does not latch properly, if you have an oversupply of milk, or if you go too long between feedings or pumpings.

- Pressure on the breast: Wearing tight clothing or a poorly fitting bra, sleeping on your stomach, or carrying a heavy bag on one shoulder can all put pressure on your breasts and contribute to plugged ducts.

- Stress or fatigue: Stress and fatigue can weaken your immune system and make you more susceptible to infections, including those that can lead to plugged ducts.

- Illness or injury: Mastitis, a common breastfeeding infection, can also lead to plugged ducts. In addition, any injury to the breast, such as a blow or a bruise, can cause a duct to become blocked.

Symptoms of Plugged Ducts

Plugged ducts can be uncomfortable and painful, but they are usually not serious. Common symptoms of plugged ducts include:

- A small, hard lump in the breast
- Redness and tenderness in the affected area
- Pain or discomfort while breastfeeding

- A feeling of fullness or heaviness in the breast
- Flu-like symptoms, such as fever or chills

If you are experiencing any of these symptoms, it is important to address the issue promptly to prevent it from developing into a more serious condition, such as mastitis.

Relieving Plugged Ducts

There are several effective strategies for relieving plugged ducts and restoring comfort to your breastfeeding experience. Here are some tips to help you effectively manage plugged ducts:

- Nurse frequently: The best way to prevent and relieve plugged ducts is to nurse your baby frequently and ensure that your breasts are fully drained at each feeding. Make sure your baby is latching properly and offer both breasts at each feeding to help prevent milk from accumulating in the ducts.

- Apply heat: Applying a warm compress to the affected breast can help to loosen the blockage and promote milk flow. You can use a warm washcloth, a heating pad, or take a warm shower to help relieve the pain and discomfort of plugged ducts.

- Massage the affected area: Gently massaging the lump in a circular motion towards the nipple can help to break up the blockage and facilitate milk flow. You can also try using a breast pump or hand expressing to help remove the blockage.

- Change positions: Experimenting with different breastfeeding positions can help to ensure that all areas of the breast are effectively drained. Try nursing your baby in a reclined position or using a side-lying position to help encourage milk flow and relieve plugged ducts.

- Stay hydrated and well-nourished: Drinking plenty of water and eating a balanced diet can help to support your overall health and immune system, making you less susceptible to infections and plugged ducts.

- Rest and relax: Stress and fatigue can weaken your immune system and make you more prone to infections, so it is important to prioritize self-care and relaxation. Take time to rest and recharge, and ask for help from friends and family members if needed.

When to Seek Help

In most cases, plugged ducts can be effectively relieved at home with the strategies outlined above. However, if you are experiencing severe pain, a high fever, or if your symptoms are not improving despite your efforts, it is important to seek help from a healthcare provider. These may be signs of a more serious condition, such as mastitis, that requires medical attention.

In addition, if you are experiencing recurrent plugged ducts or if you have concerns about your breastfeeding experience, consider reaching out to a lactation consultant for support and guidance.

Conclusion

In the journey of motherhood, few challenges are as daunting as the discomfort of plugged ducts disrupting the beautiful bond between you and your little one. Yet, within the pages of "**From Discomfort to Relief: A Holistic Approach to Clearing Plugged Ducts Naturally**," you've discovered a beacon of hope and empowerment.

Throughout this journey, we've explored gentle yet effective natural remedies and self-care practices designed to alleviate the discomfort of plugged ducts and restore harmony to your breastfeeding experience. From soothing herbal compresses to gentle massage techniques, each strategy is a testament to the power of holistic healing in nurturing both body and spirit.

But beyond the practical solutions lies a deeper truth: the journey from discomfort to relief is not just about finding physical comfort—it's about reclaiming your power as a mother. It's about embracing the wisdom of your body and trusting in its innate ability to heal. It's about honoring the sacred bond between you and your little one, and nurturing it with love and compassion.

As you close the final chapter of this book, remember this: you are not alone in your journey. Countless mothers have faced similar struggles and emerged stronger on the other side. Your experience is a testament to your resilience and dedication to providing the best for your child.

So, dear reader, carry with you the wisdom gleaned from these pages as you continue your journey of motherhood. Let the gentle remedies and self-care practices serve as your allies, guiding you towards a more comfortable and fulfilling breastfeeding experience.

May you find solace in the embrace of natural healing, and may your journey from discomfort to relief be filled with grace and resilience. Here's to embracing the holistic approach and nurturing yourself and your little one with love, compassion, and unwavering determination.

Biography

Meet Alice Brendan, a passionate advocate for women's health and holistic wellness. With a background in lactation consulting and a deep understanding of the challenges faced by breastfeeding mothers, Alice is the driving force behind " **From Discomfort to Relief: Natural Remedies and Self-Care Practices for Plugged Ducts.**"

Drawing from her extensive expertise and personal experiences, Alice's mission is to empower women who suffer from duct problems when breastfeeding, as well as those who seek to prevent these challenges altogether.

Her compassionate approach to healing encompasses not only physical remedies but also the importance of self-care and nurturing the mind, body, and spirit.

Beyond her professional pursuits, Alice finds joy in connecting with nature and exploring new cultures through travel. Whether she's hiking through scenic trails or immersing herself in the vibrant tapestry of a foreign market, Alice's curiosity and zest for life shine through in all she does.

With " **From Discomfort to Relief**: Natural Remedies and Self-Care Practices for Plugged Ducts," Alice invites readers to embark on a journey of healing and empowerment.

Through her enthusiastic guidance and heartfelt wisdom, she seeks to uplift and inspire women to embrace natural remedies and self-care practices, fostering a more harmonious and fulfilling breastfeeding experience.

Join Alice on this transformative journey and discover the power of holistic healing to bring comfort and relief to your life. Here's to embracing wellness, one gentle step at a time, with Alice Brendan as your trusted guide.